Cosmetic Injectable Fillers

Editor

COREY S. MAAS

FACIAL PLASTIC SURGERY CLINICS OF NORTH AMERICA

www.facialplastic.theclinics.com

Consulting Editor
J. REGAN THOMAS

November 2015 • Volume 23 • Number 4

ELSEVIER

1600 John F. Kennedy Boulevard • Suite 1800 • Philadelphia, Pennsylvania, 19103-2899

http://www.theclinics.com

FACIAL PLASTIC SURGERY CLINICS OF NORTH AMERICA Volume 23, Number 4
November 2015 ISSN 1064-7406, ISBN-13: 978-0-323-41330-5

Editor: Jessica McCool
Developmental Editor: Alison Swety

Facial Plastic Surgery Clinics of North America (ISSN 1064-7406) is published quarterly by Elsevier Inc., 360 Park Avenue South, New York, NY 10010-1710. Months of issue are February, May, August, and November. Business and Editorial Offices: 1600 John F. Kennedy Blvd., Suite 1800, Philadelphia, PA 19103-2899. Periodicals postage paid at New York, NY, and additional mailing offices. Subscription prices are $390.00 per year (US individuals), $525.00 per year (US institutions), $445.00 per year (Canadian individuals), $653.00 per year (Canadian institutions), $535.00 per year (foreign individuals), $653.00 per year (foreign institutions), $185.00 per year (US students), and $255.00 per year (foreign students). Foreign air speed delivery is included in all *Clinics* subscription prices. All prices are subject to change without notice. POSTMASTER: Send address changes to *Facial Plastic Surgery Clinics*, Elsevier Health Sciences Division, Subscription Customer Service, 3251 Riverport Lane, Maryland Heights, MO 63043. **Customer service: 1-800-654-2452 (US and Canada); 1-314-447-8871 (outside US and Canada); Fax: 314-447-8029; E-mail: journalscustomerservice-usa@elsevier.com (for print support); journalsonline support-usa@elsevier.com (for online support).**

Reprints. For copies of 100 or more of articles in this publication, please contact the Commercial Reprints Department, Elsevier Inc., 360 Park Avenue South, New York, NY 10010-1710. Tel.: 212-633-3874; Fax: 212-633-3820; E-mail: reprints@elsevier.com.

Facial Plastic Surgery Clinics of North America is covered in *MEDLINE/PubMed (Index Medicus).*

Contributors

CONSULTING EDITOR

J. REGAN THOMAS, MD, FACS
Professor and Chairman, Department of
Otolaryngology, University of Illinois at
Chicago, Chicago, Illinois

EDITOR

COREY S. MAAS, MD, FACS
The Maas Clinic–San Francisco, Reno-Tahoe,
Associate Clinical Professor, University of
California, San Francisco, San Francisco,
California

AUTHORS

LAWRENCE S. BASS, MD, FACS
Bass Plastic Surgery, PLCC, New York,
New York

STEVEN L. BASTA, BA
CEO Tigercat Pharma, Former CEO BioForm
Medical and Merz Aesthetics, Menlo Park,
California

ANDREW BREITHAUPT, MD
Assistant Clinical Instructor, Department of
Medicine, David Geffen School of Medicine,
University of California, Los Angeles, Los
Angeles, California

REBECCA FITZGERALD, MD
Assistant Clinical Instructor, Department of
Medicine, David Geffen School of Medicine,
University of California, Los Angeles, Los
Angeles, California

JACQUELINE J. GREENE, MD
Resident, Department of Otolaryngology -
Head and Neck Surgery, Northwestern
University, Chicago, Illinois

JOHN H. JOSEPH, MD
Director, Clinical Testing of Beverly Hills;
Assistant Clinical Professor, Department of
Head and Neck Surgery, University of
California, Los Angeles, Beverly Hills, California

TANYA KHAN, MD
Duke University Medical Center, Durham,
North Carolina

JOHN MARTIN, MD
Duke University Medical Center, Coral Gables,
Florida

AMIR MORADI, MD
Private Practice, Vista, California

AVA SHAMBAN, MD
AVA MD Santa Monica – Medical and
Cosmetic Dermatology, Santa Monica,
California

DOUGLAS M. SIDLE, MD, FACS
Assistant Professor, Department of
Otolaryngology - Head and Neck Surgery,
Northwestern University, Chicago, Illinois

JEFFREY WATSON, MD
University of California San Diego Medical
Center, San Diego, California

JULIE WOODWARD, MD
Duke University Medical Center, Durham,
North Carolina

Contents

The cosmetic filler industry has evolved substantially over the last 30 years. The market is characterized by multiple fillers and a competitive dynamic among major aesthetics companies. Marketing in the United States and Europe has been different owing to regulatory constraints. Differences have led to more rapid growth in the European market. The US market has evolved owing to growth of major companies with multiple product portfolios and leverage in consumer promotion and aesthetics office marketing owing to scale. The evolution of the filler market will include new materials, injection techniques, and facilitation devices, and new areas of injection.

This article is a detailed summary of the device tissue interface regarding cosmetic injectable fillers, specifically focusing on hyaluronic acid fillers. Hyaluronic acid-injectable fillers are used extensively for soft tissue volumizing and contouring. Many different hyaluronic acid-injectable fillers are available on the market and differ in terms of hyaluronic acid concentration, particle size, cross-linking density, requisite needle size, duration, stiffness, hydration, presence of lidocaine, type of cross-linking technology, and cost. Although much is known about how the devices interact with biologic tissues and how they produce their effects, they continue to be actively studied for tissue engineering purposes. The biomechanical and biochemical effects of HA on the local microenvironment of the injected site are key to its success as a soft tissue filler. Knowledge of the tissue device interface will help guide the facial practitioner and lead to optimal outcomes for patients.

There are several different classes of synthetic dermal fillers and volume enhancers including semipermanent and permanent products available in the United States. Based on clinical and scientific evidence, this article reviews the chemical and polymeric properties, clinical data, patient selection, indications for use, injection technique, and adverse event profiles of permanent synthetic injectables currently used in clinical practice in the United States: medical-grade liquid injectable silicone and polymethyl methacrylate. Understanding the unique characteristics of these two products reinforces the advantages and disadvantages of each, including under what circumstances they should be used and why they perform the way they do.

The use of facial fillers has greatly expanded over the past several years. Along with increased use comes a rise in documented complications, ranging from poor cosmetic result to nodules, granulomas, necrosis, and blindness. Awareness of the potential types of complications and options for management, in addition to the underlying facial anatomy, are imperative to delivering the best patient care. This article defines the complications and how to treat them and provides suggestions to avoid serious adverse outcomes.

 Videos of dorsal hand treatment with calcium hydroxyl appetite; and panfacial treatment with poly-L-lactic acid accompany this article

Over the last decade, many studies of the structural changes observed in the aging face (in bone, fat pads, facial ligaments, muscle, skin) have increased our understanding that facial rejuvenation is more complex and nuanced than simply filling lines and folds or cutting and lifting soft tissue and skin. This, in addition to the many new products introduced to the marketplace over the same period, has fueled the evolution of panfacial rejuvenation and restoration using fillers. This article discusses current techniques used with calcium hydroxylapatite and poly-L-lactic acid to safely and effectively address changes observed in the aging face.

Creating a refreshed, best version of an individual face requires knowledge of facial anatomy, understanding of the interactions of fillers and neurotoxins with tissue and muscle, and dedication to the primary principal of aesthetic responsibility. The forehead ages in a similar fashion to the rest of the face with loss of volume in both subcutaneous fat and bone. Different injection techniques are recommended for the forehead, midface, lip, and lower face. Although we understand the changes associated with aging from a global perspective, each individual ages at his or her own pace and in consideration to their specific anatomy.

Multiple fillers are available: various hyaluronic acid products, calcium hydroxylapatite, and a few others that are biocompatible with good duration and a variety of mechanical properties allowing intradermal, subdermal, and supraperiosteal injection. Facial features can be reshaped with great control using these fillers. Aging changes, including facial volume loss, can be well-corrected. These treatments have become a mainstay of rejuvenation in the early facial aging patient. Injection technique is critical to obtaining excellent results. Threading, fanning, crosshatching, bleb, and pillar techniques must be mastered. Technical execution can only measure up to, but not exceed, the quality of the aesthetic analysis.

When evaluating the face in thirds, the upper face, midface, and lower face, one may assume the temple, midface, and lateral mandible as the pillars of these subdivisions. Many of our facial aesthetic procedures address these regions, including the lateral brow lift, midface lift, and lateral face lift. As the use of facial fillers has advanced, more emphasis is placed on the correction of the temples, midlateral face, and lateral jaw line. This article is dedicated to these facial aesthetic pillars.

FACIAL PLASTIC SURGERY CLINICS OF NORTH AMERICA

THE CLINICS ARE AVAILABLE ONLINE!
Access your subscription at:
www.theclinics.com

Preface

The New Paradigm in Facial Rejuvenation: Soft Tissue Fillers 2015

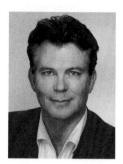

Corey S. Maas, MD, FACS

Editor

The history of cosmetic injections has seen dramatic swings in acceptance, application, and use. From the reports of fat injection by Peer in the 1950s, to nearly 20 years of exclusivity of bovine and subsequently human collagen, to our current market including a palette of molecules and materials for injection, providers in esthetics are now challenged to provide the correct product for each indication in each individual. That, remarkably, is a new paradigm. These are the primary categories for contemporary use of cosmetic injections: volume enhancement or replacement, enhancement of certain beauty features (eg, lips, chin, nose), and the softening of sharp transitions that result from aging. The latter is often thought of as the primary use of cosmetic injectable fillers as reflected in the common FDA approval pathway of nasolabial region softening of the cheek-lip transition zone, although this applies to many areas such as the labiomandibular groove and sulcus, suborbital grooves, and hollows commonly referred to as the tear trough depression and the orbital malar groove, and the genio mandibular sulcus.

It is clear from social observation, however, that the use of these products in many cases

has "gone too far" with extraordinary posttreatment lip morphology and overly bloated-looking faces that do greater harm than benefit to the patient, the physician and specialty reputation, and ultimately, the products. Industry, professional societies, and responsible thought-leaders have a duty to collaborate and bring clear standards of care to the forefront that focus on beauty and restoration that are natural and complimentary to the diverse population of patients being treated. The directive of each of the authors in this issue was to bring their unique and expert perspective to both the outstanding potential for proper use of cosmetic injectable materials and the sad reality of what appears to be at least a decade of overinflated faces and in many cases facial features that are disproportionate to the point of deformity. Clearly, a balance is needed in treating the face, hands, and other areas of potential indication between restoring volume and managing the skin envelope. The advances in nonsurgical skin tightening have provided some tools for these purposes, and thoughtful practitioners provide or refer for surgical restoration of the skin

Facial Plast Surg Clin N Am 23 (2015) ix–x
http://dx.doi.org/10.1016/j.fsc.2015.09.001
1064-7406/15/$ – see front matter © 2015 Published by Elsevier Inc.

envelope. Surgical implants, skin repositioning, and feature balancing remain integral to the paradigm with thoughtful use of cosmetic injection as described by our expert authors. I would like to extend a special thanks to each of them and to Steven L. Basta for providing an industry perspective on this rapidly expanding service line. Beauty is our business. Natural beauty should be the goal.

Corey S. Maas, MD, FACS
The Maas Clinic–
San Francisco, Reno-Tahoe
University of California
San Francisco
2400 Clay Street
San Francisco, CA 94115, USA

E-mail address:
drmaas@maasclinic.com

Cosmetic Fillers
Perspectives on the Industry

Steven L. Basta, BA

KEYWORDS

- Dermal filler • Cosmetic filler • Industry • Filler market • Injectables market

KEY POINTS

- The cosmetic filler market is characterized by multiple filler materials of varying performance characteristics designed for application in different areas of the face, and by competitive dynamics among major aesthetics companies.
- Marketing in the United States and Europe has been quite different owing to regulatory constraints in the US market, leading to more rapid growth in the European market.
- The US market has evolved significantly in recent years driven by scale and consumer marketing strength among major companies with multiple product portfolios.
- The evolution of the filler market will include new materials, injection techniques, and facilitation devices, and new areas of injection.

EVOLUTION OF THE FILLER MARKET

In the 1980s, the introduction of collagen heralded a new era of minimally invasive aesthetic procedures. In the early days of collagen, some industry analysts estimated the entire dermal filler market could potentially be $40 million in product revenue eventually. Women could hardly imagine getting injections regularly for aesthetic enhancement, and no one could foresee injecting a toxin in the face regularly throughout one's adult life. Needless to say, the aesthetics business has come a long way since then.

In the 1990s, collagen continued to dominate the US filler market, whereas internationally the hyaluronic acid (HA) fillers emerged as the new leaders in the market owing to longevity, performance, and handling advantages versus collagen. Permanent fillers were also introduced in the 1990s in Europe with mixed results. The introduction of HA resulted in rapid growth and differentiation in the filler business in Europe, well before similar improvements were available in the United States.

The launch of Cosmoplast and Cosmederm in the United States expanded the market by eliminating skin testing, but lacked the durability improvement of the HAs. In the filler market, 2003 proved to be a transformative year. The market for dermal fillers expanded profoundly with the approval and launch of Restylane, which offered superior augmentation in a single syringe as compared with a single syringe of collagen. As patient satisfaction improved, and the wave of beauty magazines highlighted Restylane as the best new thing from Europe, adoption of Restylane far exceeded the anticipated level, and approximately doubled the peak adoption of collagen in the first year.

Along with the launch of Restylane, the introduction of other forms of HA, plus new materials such as Radiesse and Sculptra, drove rapid growth in the aesthetics market. The range of products on offer provided a range of lifting and volumizing

Disclosure: Mr S.L. Basta served as CEO of BioForm Medical 2002–2010 and served as CEO of Merz Aesthetics 2010–2011. Mr. S.L. Basta currently serves as CEO of Tigercat Pharma, a pharmaceutical development company developing a therapy for chronic pruritus. Mr S.L. Basta has no current affiliations with any of the aesthetics companies or products described in this article.
590 Berkeley Avenue, Menlo Park, CA 94025, USA
E-mail address: sbasta100@gmail.com

Facial Plast Surg Clin N Am 23 (2015) 417–421
http://dx.doi.org/10.1016/j.fsc.2015.07.001

characteristics; some offered perceived greater longevity than Restylane. The market rapidly segmented based on duration and handling characteristics. Duration is often cited as the differentiation factor, because it is easy to reference a number to describe a product as a "3-month," "6-month," or "12-month" filler. Such labels derived from several factors, including (i) the ease of describing a product based on duration versus the complexity of describing distinctions in handling properties, viscosity, injection effect, and so on, (ii) the desire for companies to be able to differentiate their fillers, and (iii) US Food and Drug Administration (FDA) restrictions on marketing claims, which constrained the ability to describe handling differences to clinicians in terms that implied different clinical outcomes.

Why the United States' and European Union Filler Markets are Different: Regulatory Drivers and History

The regulatory constraints of seeking FDA approval and the limitations on FDA-compliant marketing cause the differences between the United States and the European Union (EU) filler markets. Four key constraints in the US regulatory environment drove the historical US market approval lag and lack of competitive differentiation relative to filler marketing in Europe. These constraints are:

1. Premarket approval requirements in the United States for many years constrained fillers to an approval indication of "moderate to severe lines and wrinkles" and directed all the companies to run comparative trials against collagen. The most confident path to approval for any filler company was to run a direct comparison study against collagen (because it is relatively straightforward statistically to run a noninferiority study against a known weaker competitor). This resulted in the new product approvals for Restylane, Juvederm, Radiesse, Artefill, and other products all demonstrating noninferiority to collagen to get exactly the same approval indication.
2. Making superiority or differential effect claims in the United States is a high hurdle. For example, BioForm performed comparative trials of Radiesse in Europe against Restylane and Juvederm and could use those data in Europe, but the US approval trials were conducted against collagen, so that the comparative data against HA are not in the United States product approval labeling, limiting how it can be used in marketing materials. FDA marketing standards intended to protect patients and physicians from false claims have the unintended consequence in the US filler market of hampering communications that would serve to provide differentiation information. Thus, the marketing of fillers in the US market for many years was restricted to very similar nasolabial fold claims showing similar before and after pictures.
3. The FDA has been focused on correction of defects or disease, and has been much less receptive to enhancement claims. That is what drives a lines/wrinkles focus of filler approvals. It also leads to acne scar or facial lipoatrophy indications. Lip augmentation or facial enhancement, by contrast, is slower to work through the FDA approval process because it is not correcting a deficit. That requirement limits the ability to get more superficial fillers or specifically designed lip fillers through the FDA approval process and limits the range of different fillers available to US physicians.
4. The time and cost of US-approval trials limit the range of fillers available. In the EU, by some estimates more than 50 forms of HA are available, ranging from very light materials designed for middermal injection for superficial wrinkles, to very viscous materials for facial contouring through larger gauge needles. The range of materials in the US market is limited by the need to demonstrate effectiveness of each form of material in the target indication. The trials take several years, and the full approval cycle including manufacturing validations, clinical studies, preclinical studies, and so on can be $10 to $30 million and 3 to 7 years per clinical product form developed. There is diminishing marketing return to the third, fourth, or fifth form of a filler approved within a family of fillers. The time required and cost of developing subsequent forms of fillers in Europe can be 10% to 20% of the US development cost.

Certainly, there is now evolution beyond the lines and wrinkles indication after 30 years of filler development in the United States. The approvals of Sculptra and Radiesse for facial lipoatrophy and the more recent FDA reviews of hand augmentation, acne scars, and facial volume indications for various products open the clinical path to new indications.

The EU filler market provides a completely different competitive profile. By 2010, more than 50 distinct fillers were on the market in several European countries. Counting all the derivative forms and modified viscosities, the number may be much greater now. The US market at the time had fewer than 10 actively marketed fillers. The market in Europe evolved in a regulatory climate in which demonstrating short-term safety with relatively moderate work was the hurdle to market entry.

The marketing ability in Europe to promote indications with relatively modest trials meant that fillers could be positioned for lips, contouring, lipoatrophy, hands, and other age-related volume loss effects beyond the lines and wrinkles indication in the United States. Fillers in Europe can be marketed for lip fullness and for vermilion border applications. Fillers can be marketed for superficial injection or for volume enhancement and facial shaping.

Good and bad consequences come from the regulatory differences. The downside to the lower regulatory hurdles in some cases was that less safe fillers were introduced. The upside was dramatic growth in the EU filler market and the ability of physicians to provide patients with better outcomes. The EU filler market is significantly larger and has been for many years than the EU aesthetic neurotoxin market. The inverse is true in the United States. This distinction results largely from regulatory differences, as noted.

THE BATTLE FOR YOUR ATTENTION AND THAT OF YOUR STAFF

A ground war of sorts has emerged in all filler markets worldwide. This is a battle for space in the front office, in the treatment rooms, and in the hearts, minds, and most important habits of every aesthetics office staff member and filler injector. The major filler companies rapidly expanded their sales organizations to influence each aesthetics practice to convert patients or adopt their fillers. By 2010, the sales teams consisted of more than 500 representatives for these 4 companies in the US market. That is 1 representative for every 20 or so major injector practices. You may see a representative in your practice almost every day if you have a busy aesthetics practice.

The relationship between an aesthetics company and a physician (or more broadly a physician's office) is complex and reflects numerous levels of symbiosis. Companies view physicians as advisors, partners, and customers, all of which one would expect. However, the companies also view the physicians' office as a store front to be tailored to sell their inventory, and view the physician's office staff very much as an extension of the companies' own sales teams. The ground war of competition among the aesthetics companies exists at every step through the office.

First Impressions: The Reception Area

Before a patient sees the physician to discuss a treatment, there are numerous opportunities to influence the choice of filler at every step in the office and at every touch point with the patient. The battle in the filler market involves every table in a waiting room, the back of every examination room door, and influencing the thoughts, preferences and recommendation of every member of the office staff. Anyone who talks to a patient can influence the choice.

Primacy matters greatly. A patient's first signal of which filler to use could come from the phone call to schedule the appointment or the window cling as they approach the office. What brochures you allow in your waiting room, and what training your receptionist receives, is critical to driving what fillers and other products you will actually use in your practice. You may think your patient is requesting Juvederm because that is what they really want, but they may have first heard of it from your receptionist. Just for example, a Radiesse injector once conducted her own in-house comparison of Radiesse and an HA filler and decided she wanted to use Radiesse more often for certain nasolabial folds. However, her staff, unaware of that preference, was only familiar with Restylane. For several months, every patient who called in for smile lines was scheduled for a Restylane injection, and before the patient got to the treatment room, a syringe of Restylane was pulled from the shelf. The choice of filler to be used in that office was not driven by the patient or by the injector, but rather by habit of the receptionist who was only aware that the office had Restylane.

The Office Staff and Patient Influencers

In the office, the patient selection of a filler product relates to numerous variables:

- Who advises or asks the patient about areas of concern, treatment, product alternatives, and other aspects of the visit and the relationship?
- Is there a discussion of an overall plan with the physician, an aesthetician, an office business manager, or a patient coordinator?

For example, if a patient wishes to get certain areas corrected that could be treated with fillers or a toxin, but other areas also need correction, some offices manage this conversation with a broad treatment discussion by the physician, and then a budget discussion by another staff member. This can be an opportunity to pitch value messages associated with longevity of certain products, or efficiency, or to establish a recurring revenue model with frequent follow-up visits. In the best practices, this economic conversation happens with a purposeful structure. The filler companies are fully engaged (if the sales representative is doing their job well) at driving that conversation with the key patient influencer toward use of their fillers and now, with consolidation, toward their portfolio of facial aesthetics products. This ground war in filler marketing happens beyond the discussions and focus of the physician at times, and can have a profound impact on practice adoption and use.

A perhaps surprising amount of focus at the filler companies is not on the physician, but on the office staff and every patient touch point. Many physicians may perceive themselves to select fillers for their patients or may perceive that they are providing patients "what the patient wants." However, the patients do not know what they want or need; they are influenced throughout the practice by every touch point, and those touch points are the primary field of competition of the aesthetics companies.

Injector Confidence

A filler will not be injected by a physician/injector who is not comfortable and confident using it. The physician or nurse injector is necessarily the single most important element of the sales channel for obvious reasons. If the person injecting a filler is not confident with a particular product, nothing else matters. The rapid adoption of HA fillers in the United States reflects several factors that drove injector confidence:

- Restylane was already the number 1 filler in Europe when launched in the United States
- HA is reversible.
- Lower volume syringe formats make the product feel softer and smoother, creating less perception of significant impact.

Confidence means a lot when picking up a syringe. In the early days after Radiesse approved for aesthetic, physician uncertainty was the single greatest hurdle to adoption. BioForm's investment in a nationwide team of clinical trainers to spend time in physicians' offices was directed toward meeting this confidence imperative.

PATIENT CHOICE INFLUENCE

Juvederm became the number 1 filler in the US market within 2 years of launch. For a decade before the US launch, Juvederm was number 2

in Europe to the Restylane line of HA fillers. What changed? Allergan launched Juvederm with a 250-person sales organization, more than twice that of any competitor, with the leverage of Botox volume-based bundling and incentives, and with significant of direct-to-consumer advertising. The effect was to grow the total US filler market substantially and to move market perception and habit quickly from Restylane to Juvederm for many procedures.

Many physicians indicate that the path of least resistance and highest patient satisfaction is to "give the patient what they ask for." In that environment, direct-to-consumer marketing and the ability to drive consumers to specific providers creates enormous leverage in the aesthetics market. A leading Radiesse customer whose use of the product declined with the launch of Juvederm once told me, "I have to use Juvederm more to maintain my Botox.com status. That's where I get many of my patients." This power of the aesthetics companies to drive patient referrals has driven a dramatic shift in the nature of the marketplace battle and will drive future consolidation of the business.

The cost of creating patient awareness of a new aesthetics product is high, and the leverage of putting it through an existing sales and marketing infrastructure is even higher. The cross-selling leverage of programs like the Allergan points pyramid for aesthetics practices or the Brilliant Distinctions rewards program for consumers creates new product introduction leverage. If a patient's Botox is less expensive because they use Juvederm, it becomes much harder for a smaller company to introduce a comparable HA filler to Juvederm.

A FEW THOUGHTS ON POSSIBLE FUTURE DEVELOPMENTS IN THE INDUSTRY
Consolidation

Consolidation to a few, large players has already emerged as a core feature of the aesthetics market. The cost of building a sales team with more than 100 members to reach aesthetics customers may be prohibitive for the launch today of a single filler company, as we did with BioForm nearly 10 years ago. The landscape of competition will be set by multiple companies that each have several good fillers (or more), a neurotoxin, and possibly several topicals or other differentiating products in the portfolio.

New Ways to Inject

The European market has started to see the introduction of injection assist devices. As fillers become more viscous, or need to be injected in greater volumes, assist devices may overcome the injection pressure challenge. If fillers are used over large surface areas for dermal hydration, for example to rejuvenate the neck or chest or mitigate superficial wrinkles, new injection devices that achieve intradermal injection more easily may be important. Precision of injection depth and amounts may become quite important and be facilitated by technology improvements.

New Areas to Inject

The EU filler market as described may give foreshadowing clues to the US market. In that respect, the evolution of fillers for volume enhancement and facial contouring is more advanced in Europe than in the United States. This may be a powerful long-term trend, as a core facial change that marks aging is lost volume. The US approval of Voluma complements the growing use of Radiesse and Sculptra over several years in volume applications. However, many filler injectors in the United States have been slower to integrate volume injection procedures and contouring procedures into their practices. This author believes that this trend is largely driven by the marketing of fillers in the United States for lines and wrinkles, rather than as in Europe for volume restoration and for a range of applications based on the properties of the fillers. The face loses volume over time, and restoring volume and shape will prove to be more impactful than filling lines for many patients. Hand and acne scar indications highlight the breadth of filler market growth opportunities and the fact that physicians may find ways to enhance aesthetics in many areas with either large amounts of viscous fillers or small amounts of appropriately targeted fillers to create beautiful aesthetic improvements.

New Materials

Many have speculated about which is the perfect filler material. There is no perfect filler. What is needed in the lips (flow characteristics, feel, etc) is different from what is needed in the cheek. What is needed for a patient with superficial marionette lines is different from the 80-year-old patients with severe folds that needs many areas corrected. The fillers we have today are very good, but there are significant gaps in the portfolio. Future fillers may improve significantly with materials that may change property after injection, so that they are easy to inject in liquid state, and then become more solid for contouring applications. Such products have been tested, some modified by temperature upon injection, and some by application of lasers. There may be long-term fillers to come in the future that overcome the safety questions of permanent fillers by being reversible or through other means of mitigating reactions. The combination of fillers and energy devices or fillers and active agents that accelerate tissue growth could herald a new wave of facial rejuvenation products that actually cause replenishment of facial tissues or remodeling and rejuvenation of skin over time to truly reverse the effects of age and gravity.

SUMMARY

The dermal filler market has rapidly evolved in the United States over the past 12 years and in Europe over the past 20. From the early days of collagen to the introduction of multiple forms of HA to the development of a range of fillers using multiple materials, the market has provided tools to physicians that delight patients and provide the opportunity for a terrific aesthetics practice. The industry will continue to get stronger, to drive patients to your practice, and to provide you tools that produce great outcomes.

The Hyaluronic Acid Fillers
Current Understanding of the Tissue Device Interface

Jacqueline J. Greene, MD, Douglas M. Sidle, MD*

KEYWORDS

- Injectable fillers • HA fillers • Hyaluronic acid • Cosmetic injectables • Tissue device interface

KEY POINTS

- Hyaluronic acid-injectable fillers are used extensively for soft tissue volumizing and contouring.
- Many different hyaluronic acid-injectable fillers are available on the market and differ in terms of hyaluronic acid concentration, particle size, cross-linking density, requisite needle size, duration, stiffness, hydration, presence of lidocaine, type of cross-linking technology, and cost.
- Hyaluronic acid is a natural component of many soft tissues, is identical across species minimizing immunogenicity has been linked to wound healing and skin regeneration, and is currently actively being studied for tissue engineering purposes. The biomechanical and biochemical effects of HA on the local microenvironment of the injected site are key to its success as a soft tissue filler. Knowledge of the tissue device interface will help guide the facial practitioner and lead to optimal outcomes for patients.

INTRODUCTION

The use of cosmetic injectables, including collagen, hyaluronic acid (HA), fat, synthetic polymers (polylactic acid, polymethylmethacrylate), and calcium hydroxyapatite, has significantly increased in popularity over the past 2 decades. The American Society of Plastic Surgeons reports an increase from 652,888 soft tissue filler procedures in 2000 to 2.3 million in 2014, whereas more invasive surgical procedures have become slightly less popular (the number of facelifts have decreased by 4% from 2000 to 2014).[1] HA has become the top injected soft filler agent around the world (1.8 million procedures reported in 2014[1]). The goal of this report is to investigate the rapid transition from other soft tissue fillers to HA following US Food and Drug Administration (FDA) approval and the interesting biomechanical and biochemical advantages behind this immensely popular biomaterial.

Early biomedical applications of HA were quite diverse, including joint synovial fluid replacement to treat osteoarthritis[2] and in ophthalmologic surgery as a vitreous replacement and for retinal detachment surgeries.[3] In 1994, Ghersetich and colleagues[4] reported decreased skin HA content with aging. HA-based dermal fillers were first available in 1996 in Europe,[5] but the first HA cosmetic injectable was not approved by the FDA in the United States until 2003 with the approval of Restylane (Q-Med, Uppsala, Sweden) followed by Hylaform in 2004 (Genzyme [now Allergan], Santa

Disclosures: The authors have no financial or other conflicts of interest to disclose.
Department of Otolaryngology - Head and Neck Surgery, Northwestern University, 676 N. St. Clair, Suite 1325, Chicago, IL 60611, USA
* Corresponding author. Facial Plastic and Reconstructive Surgery, Department of Otolaryngology - Head and Neck Surgery, Northwestern University, 675 North Saint Clair Street, Suite 15-200, Chicago, IL 60611.
E-mail address: dsidle@nm.org

Facial Plast Surg Clin N Am 23 (2015) 423–432
http://dx.doi.org/10.1016/j.fsc.2015.07.002
1064-7406/15/$ – see front matter © 2015 Elsevier Inc. All rights reserved.

Barbara, CA, USA). HA injectable fillers have been used as dermal fillers to restore soft tissue loss from aging in a variety of sites from the nasolabial folds, temporal fossa, malar fat pads, marionette lines, lip augmentation, and glabellar lines. They have also been used to correct the lipoatrophy associated with human immunodeficiency virus[6] and for vocal fold augmentation.[7] HA has also been studied as a skin-rejuvenating agent in mesotherapy, which involves multiple microinjections into the skin dermis for skin rejuvenation.[8]

Significantly, HA fillers were approved by the FDA as a device rather than a drug, which helped hasten its approval in the United States. One of the criteria by which the FDA defines a medical device is "the intent to affect the structure or any function of the body of man or other animals, and which does not achieve its primary intended purposes through chemical action within or on the body of man or other animals and which is not dependent upon being metabolized for the achievement of any of its primary intended purposes."[9] Indeed, the biomechanical effects of HA on the local microenvironment of the injected site are key to its success as a soft tissue filler. HA fillers have additional interesting properties beyond simple volumizing agents; they have been shown to increase collagen production in the local environment as well as change the fibroblast morphology.[10–12]

An ideal soft tissue implant for cosmetic purposes has the following characteristics: (1) biocompatibility or low tissue reactivity; (2) minimal migration; (3) ease of applicability; (4) bioresorbability; and (5) nonteratogenicity and noncarcinogenicity.[13] HA fillers fulfill all of these requirements in that they have not been shown to bind the surrounding cells on injection, produce very little inflammatory reaction because HA is structurally identical across species, possess viscoelastic properties that allow for easy injection as well as maintenance of shape over time, and are ultimately temporary. The minimal tissue reactivity and migration properties of injected HA support the perception of HA fillers as implants and were key to FDA approval as a device. A thorough knowledge of HA biomechanics, biochemistry, manufacturing processes, and materials science properties will help guide the clinical practitioner and lead to optimal outcomes for patients.

HYALURONIC ACID STRUCTURE AND BIOCHEMISTRY

HA is a naturally occurring polymer found in the extracellular matrix of many tissues, including human hyaline cartilage, synovial joint fluid, skin dermis, brain, vitreous fluid, and soft connective tissues.[14] It is a nonsulfated glycosaminoglycan polymer consisting of alternating D-glucuronic acid and N-acetyl-D-glucosamine monosaccharide that are cross-linked into long chains.[14] Up to 30,000 of these disaccharides can be linked to form a long chain of molecular weight ranging from 10^5 to 10^7 Da that will arrange itself into a coil in aqueous solution, binding up to 1000 times its weight in water.[15] Although much of the HA found in the body residents within the extracellular matrix, some of the HA forms pericellular coats or is localized within the cell.[15] The intracellular function of HA is not yet completely understood.[15] HA has also demonstrated antiviral activity for Herpes simplex virus-1 and Coxsackievirus B5 in vitro.[16] Absence of HA has been described in mucopolysaccharidosis IX, whereas elevated serum HA has been noted in the skin of patients with Marfan, Ehlers-Danhlos syndromes, as well as several autoimmune diseases, including scleroderma, dermatomyositis, and lupus.[15] Melanoma and basal cell carcinoma cells have been found to promote HA synthesis and deposition.[15]

The distribution of HA varies with aging; for example, newborn mice epidermis contains 80 to 90 ng/mg of dry weight HA, but adult mice epidermis contains just 20 to 30 ng/mg of dry weight HA.[15] In addition, different anatomic sites contain different amounts of HA; for example, forearm skin contains twice the amount of HA as back skin.[15] HA metabolism also varies by location; within the epidermis, HA is degraded by hyaluronidase enzymes following endocytosis, whereas in the dermis, degraded HA is drained by afferent lymphatics.[15]

ROLE IN WOUND HEALING

HA may play a key role in wound healing and skin regeneration. It is theorized that scarless wound healing found in fetal skin may be due to the higher HA content compared to children or adults.[15] HA may also play different roles depending on the size of the macromolecule; in early wounds, HA is broken down into low-molecular-weight HA that promotes cytokine secretion and stimulates angiogenesis, whereas during tissue remodeling, high-molecular-weight HA promotes fibroblast and keratinocyte migration and proliferation.[15] It is not quite understood why HA cosmetic injectable fillers are so well tolerated given their known effect on wound healing, but local inflammatory reactions seem to be rare.[15] Glucocorticoids decrease the amount of HA in the epidermis, which leads to steroid-induced atrophy.[15]

MANUFACTURING

HA fillers are produced from both animal sources (rooster combs in the case of Hylaform; Biomatrix Inc, Ridgefield, NJ, USA) and nonanimal sources (*Streptococci* equine *Streptococcus equi* bacteria such as Restylane; Q-Med).[17,18] The nonanimal stabilized HA products are often referred to as nonanimal source hyaluronic acid (NASHA). Most HA injectable fillers are formed via particulate manufacturing; the exception is Juvéderm (Allergan), which is manufactured via a nonparticulate proprietary method.[19] Processing via nonparticulate or particulate manufacturing is important in that particulate HA product longevity is strongly related to particle size, whereas nonparticulate HA duration is related to cross-linking density.[19] Regarding technique, large particulate HA products will require larger-bore needles to inject (~27 gauge) rather than the smaller-bore and less painful needles (~30 gauge).[19]

HA typically has to be cross-linked to avoid rapid degradation by hyaluronidase, temperature, or free radicals,[20] and different HA fillers vary by the cross-linking density and resulting stiffness.[21] Without cross-linking, exogenous HA is degraded by the liver and has a half-life of 1 to 2 days.[22] HA fillers with a higher cross-linking density can be used for deep wrinkles, versus HA fillers with a lower cross-linking density are preferable for fine wrinkles.[21] Cross-linking of HA may be monophasic (one treatment of cross-linking), such as Belotero (Merz Aesthetics Inc, San Mateo, CA, USA) and Juvéderm, or biphasic (cross-linked twice), such as for Restylane. Different chemicals are used to cross-link HA. HA can be cross-linked chemically by 1,4-butandiol diglycidylether (BDDE), such as for Restylane and Juvéderm, or divinyl sulfone (DVS), used in Hylaform (Genzyme now Allergan) and Captique (Genzyme Corp, Cambridge, MA, USA; no longer on the market).[22] Biscarbodiimide (BCDI) is used to cross-link Elevess (renamed Hydrelle in 2010; Anika Therapeutics, Palo Alto, CA, USA), whereas 1,2,7,8-diepoxyoctane (DEO) is used to cross-link Puragen (Mentor Corp, FDA approval pending).[19] Theoretically, oral antioxidants should reduce degradation of HA by free radicals, but that has not been proven.[23]

COMMERCIALLY AVAILABLE HYALURONIC ACID INJECTABLE FILLERS IN THE UNITED STATES

Key differences among the HA injectable fillers include concentration, particle size, cross-linking density, and elastic modulus G′. Other factors to consider include cost, requisite needle size, duration, stiffness, hydration, presence of lidocaine, and type of cross-linking technology. Generally speaking, larger-particle, higher-density HA fillers are recommended for deep dermal injections, whereas smaller-particle, lower-density fillers are recommended for fine lines and wrinkles. Cross-linking may affect the longevity of the filler as well as diffusion through the skin.[24] Cross-linking HA continuously as with Belotero has been shown to produce the most homogeneous integration as compared with a monophasic cross-linking (Juvéderm) or biphasic cross-linking (Restylane).[25] The first HA filler approved by the FDA was Restylane in 2003. Since then, many HA fillers have entered the market and are summarized in **Table 1**. One new HA filler called Dermal Gel Extra or Prevelle Lift has a much larger elastic modulus than preexisting HA fillers and is similar to permanent filler materials such as hydroxyapatite; it is currently awaiting FDA approval.[26]

Most HA injectable fillers carry a low risk of infectious disease transmission or allergic reaction and generally do not require preinjection skin testing.[22] The popularity of the HA injectable fillers has led to many products being available in the United States, and choosing among them is often up to physician familiarity and preference.[27] There are few to no studies demonstrating differences in diffusion pattern and spread of the different HA fillers. An additional distinction among the commercially available HA fillers is the inclusion of lidocaine as a local anesthetic; although this may make the particular product more appealing for patients, there are concerns about diluting the HA, leading to a less concentrated filler.

COMPARISON WITH OTHER DERMAL FILLERS

Although a detailed analysis of other types of cosmetic injectable fillers are beyond the scope of this article, key advantages and disadvantages of HA compared with other dermal fillers are highlighted.

Both collagen and HA are macromolecules native to the human body, but key differences with regards to manufacturing and clinical applicability exist. Past experience with HA fillers has demonstrated that the HA is nonimmunogenic, unlike collagen, which if derived from bovine sources, may provoke an allergic or immune response.[13,28,29] This allergic or immune response is likely due to the fact that, although collagen can vary slightly between species, HA has been reported to have an identical chemical structure across species. HA injectable fillers do not require

Table 1
Summary of commercially available hyaluronic acid fillers

HA Filler	Subtype	HA Source	Cross-Linking Agent	HA Concentration (mg/mL)	% Cross-Linked HA	Particle Size (μm)	G′ (Pa)
Restylane		NASHA	BDDE	20	<1	250–300	864
	Fine Lines (Touch)	NASHA	BDDE	—	—	—	—
	Perlane (renamed Restylane Lyft June 2015)	NASHA	BDDE	20	<1	650	977
Juvéderm	Ultra	NASHA	BDDE	24	6	—	207
	Ultra Plus	NASHA	BDDE	24–30	8	—	105
	Voluma	NASHA	—	—	—	—	—
Belotero	—	NASHA	BDDE	22.5	—	—	128
Captique[a]	—	NASHA	DVS	5.5	20	500	—
Hylaform[a]	—	animal	DVS	5.5	12–20	500	100
	Plus	animal	DVS	5.5	12	700–750	140
Eleyess	(renamed Hydrelle 2010)	NASHA	BCDI	28	—	200	—
Prevelle Silk	—	NASHA	DVS	5.5	12	350	230–260
Prevelle Lift	(also known as Dermal Gel Extra)	NASHA	—	22	7	—	1800
Puragen[a]	—	NASHA	DEO	20	—	—	—

Most of these products are available with or without lidocaine.

Abbreviations: BCDI, biscarbodiimide; BDDE, 1,4-butandiol diglycidylether; DEO, 2,7,8-diepoxyoctane; DVS, divinyl sulfone; G′, storage or elastic modulus; HA, hyaluronic acid; NASHA, non-animal source HA; Pa, Pascal.

[a] Hylaform and Captique are no longer on the market; Puragen is approved in Europe but FDA approval is pending.

skin testing before use, in contrast to bovine-derived collagen fillers.[30] Some HAs have an equivalent or longer duration of efficacy compared with other nonpermanent fillers such as fat and collagen and may have a synergistic effect for even longer duration when combined with BOTOX.[22,30]

The longevity of HA fillers as compared with other dermal fillers is another important advantage. Commercially available HA fillers include Restylane (Q-Med), Juvéderm, Hylaform, and Captique and typically last at least approximately 6 months, and up to 2 years *in vivo*.[28] One clear advantage of HA fillers is the potential reversibility with the enzyme hyaluronidase[31]; other nonde-gradable or permanent injectable fillers would require surgical excision for removal. Hyaluronidase, an enzyme that specifically targets HA, is available as Vitrase (Bausch & Lomb, Rochester, NY, USA), Hyelenex (Halozyme Therapeutics, San Diego, CA, USA), and Amphadase (Amphastar Pharmaceuticals, Nanjing, China) and is typically used if the HA filler is incorrectly injected or abnormally collects or in cases of infection or granuloma formation.[30]

TISSUE DEVICE INTERFACE

Materials Science and Engineering investigates new materials from the perspectives of physics, chemistry, and engineering and stresses the paradigm that the processing and structure of these new materials are critical influences on their overall function. The biomechanical and biochemical advantages of HA fillers have led to its immense popularity over other injectable cosmetic fillers. Key properties of HA include its volumizing properties, osmotic effects, viscoelastic mechanical properties, and biochemical effects on the local cellular environment.

It has always been thought that HA fillers simply worked by occupying space and filling voids; however, further investigation has revealed that HA is not a static material. HA has a high fixed charge density that is osmotically active in that it attracts water molecules resulting in swelling, typically within the constraints of a cross-linked collagen network in normal tissue.[32] It is theorized that the natural abundance of HA within the dermis along with the lymphatic system aids in regulating water content within the dermis.[15] When injected for soft tissue augmentation, HA fillers absorb water and swell, increasing the compressive strength of the injected filler.[20,33] This swelling effect may lead to slight expansion 24 hours after correction depending on the degree of hydration of the HA filler before injection.[23] This effect has been reported

to last for 3 to 6 months depending on the site of injection (3–4-month duration is reported for lips vs 6 months for the glabellar and forehead region[22]). One study of intradermal injection of Restylane into mice demonstrated an increase in volume to 1.8 of the original size by 1 week with subsequent decrease in size over 16 weeks.[28] In another study, Restylane was injected intradermally into human volunteers, and for up to 26 weeks a small amount of the injected HA was still visible.[20]

Minimal tissue reactivity and migration of injected HA are important characteristics both for safety approval from the FDA and for prevention of scar formation or inflammation. HA likely achieves these goals through its negatively charged end carboxyl groups (COO−), which lead to poor cell-adhesion properties and thereby minimal tissue reactivity and migration.[28] One study evaluating the longevity of volumizing effect of HA injectables with MRI noted that if injected onto bone, the HA eventually formed a capsule and lengthened the duration of the filler, although these patients were seeking cosmetic volumization of craniofacial deformities such as nasal dorsum correction or frontal bone irregularities following previous neurosurgical procedures, rather than rhytid correction.[34] *In vivo* studies of HA dermal filler subcutaneous injection into mice demonstrate minimal fibroblast infiltration, rather, formation of a capsule surrounding the filler.[28] This finding is echoed in a separate article that detailed that the HA dermal filler (Restylane) simply occupied space but did not promote tissue regeneration or angiogenesis, as compared with injected gelatin spheres that were resorbed and replaced by fibrous, vascularized neodermis within 8 weeks.[20]

The volumizing and space-occupying properties of HA fillers are likely the key reasons behind its success for soft tissue augmentation; however, there are several other aspects of the HA mechanism of action that contribute to its efficacy. There are multiple studies describing that aged skin has decreased type I collagen content due to degradation by matrix metalloproteinases (collagen-cleaving enzymes).[35] A study from the University of Michigan reports an increase in type I and III collagen deposition, increased profibrotic growth factors, and a stretched appearance to fibroblasts at 4 and 13 weeks in forearm skin that was injected with NASHA in 11 volunteers.[10] The change in morphology of the fibroblasts and increased collagen deposition following NASHA injection can be seen through both routine histologic light microscopy and transmission electron microscopy in **Fig. 1**.

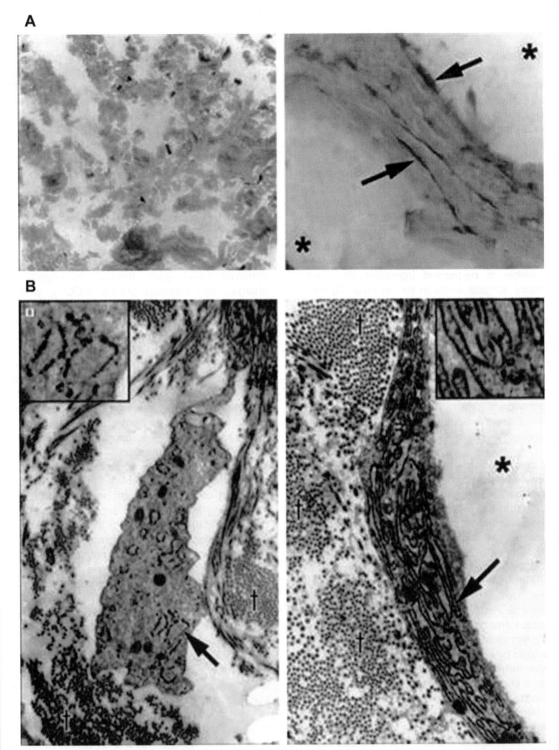

Fig. 1. Fibroblasts exhibit a stretched morphologic shape and synthetically active phenotype in skin treated with NA-SHA. Fibroblasts were visualized in skin injected with isotonic sodium chloride vehicle (*left images*) or NASHA (*right images*). Shown are representative tissue sections at 4 weeks after treatment. Open spaces (*asterisks*) in the NASHA images are consistent with areas that contained filler material. (*A*) Tissue sections were stained for the C-terminus of type I procollagen, and positively stained fibroblasts (*arrows*) appear dark red. Cell nuclei were counterstained with hematoxylin (*blue*) (original magnification, ×40). (*B*) Fibroblasts were examined with transmission electron microscopy. Daggers denote collagen fibers/fibrils in the extracellular matrix. Arrows denote rough endoplasmic reticulum, which are intracellular structures involved in synthesizing proteins, including collagen. These are shown at higher power in the insets (main panels: original magnification, ×2200; insets, ×5300). (*From* Wang F, Garza LA, Kang S, et al. *In vivo* stimulation of de novo collagen production caused by cross-linked hyaluronic acid dermal filler injections in photodamaged human skin. Arch Dermatol 2007;143(2):155–63; with permission.)

The same study demonstrated fibroblasts binding to collagen rather than to injected NASHA *in vivo* and *in vitro*, suggesting that the HA does not directly stimulate fibroblasts, rather that HA changes its local microenvironment through other means.[10] It is theorized that by mechanically stretching fibroblasts, the injected HA induces cell signaling changes on the surface of fibroblasts that ultimately lead to increased production of collagen as shown in this schematic (**Fig. 2**). Similar findings of increased type I[11] and III[12] collagen production adjacent to injected cross-linked HA have also been reported in separate studies.

The rheology (how a material flows and deforms to different mechanical stressors) of fillers is critical to overall performance and can guide clinicians in optimizing aesthetic outcomes of soft tissue augmentation depending on the area of the face in question.[36] Injectable fillers need to have a combination of mechanical properties, termed viscoelasticity; they need to be viscous enough to be easily extruded through a needle or cannula and yet elastic enough to retain their shape once implanted in the face and subjected to the mechanical stresses of facial animation and other external forces.[7,36] The mechanical properties of a material can be tested in a variety of ways; for biological materials, shear stress (external force applied parallel to a surface of a material) is often described rather than compressive stress (external force applied perpendicular to the surface of a material) because most soft biological materials are largely composed of water, which is generally incompressible by normal biological forces.[37] In addition, steady shear stress will usually damage or permanently deform a biological soft material and provide little useful biomechanical information apart from failure strain.[37] Mechanical testing that is more relevant to the repetitive stresses of facial animation is applying a small oscillating shear stress to a material between 2 rheometer plates to obtain the elastic storage shear modulus G' and the loss shear or viscosity modulus G''.[37] The elastic storage shear modulus G' for a particular oscillatory rate (most commonly 5 Hz) and strain is more commonly reported for viscoelastic gels such as HA fillers,[36,37] although often some studies lack the rate and strain information, which likely contributes to variation in the reported G' for different HA fillers.

The elastic storage shear modulus G' refers to how a material can recover its shape after an external shear mechanical force. Although cross-linking the HA leads to a stiffer gel or higher G', non-cross-linked or free HA may act as a lubricant leading to a smoother injection.[23] HA dermal fillers with a higher G' are better for volumizing or lifting deep folds or in the subperiosteal plane, whereas lower G' fillers diffuse more evenly for a softer effect and are best used superficially within the

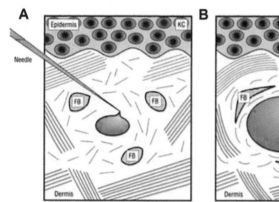
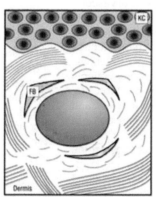
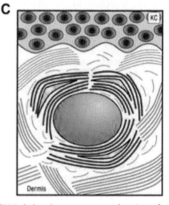

Fig. 2. Working model of mechanical tension (stretching) induced by NASHA injections as a mechanism for collagen induction in human skin. Normal skin consists of an outer epidermis composed mostly of keratinocytes (KCs), and an underlying dermis consisting mostly of extracellular matrix proteins, which are synthesized by fibroblasts (FBs). Types I and III collagen fibers are the major structural components of the extracellular matrix. In contrast to younger skin, which contains intact collagen fibers, photodamaged older skin (depicted here) contains areas of fragmented collagen fibers. (*A*) NASHA is shown as preferentially localizing in areas containing more highly fragmented collagen fibers, since these regions may be more accommodating. (*B*) This results in stretching of existing collagen fibers (*curved lines*), which is sensed by nearby fibroblasts through cell surface receptors such as integrins. In response, fibroblasts become morphologically stretched (*B*) and activated to produce extracellular matrix components (*C*), including new, intact collagen fibers (*red lines*). (*From* Wang F, Garza LA, Kang S, et al. *In vivo* stimulation of de novo collagen production caused by cross-linked hyaluronic acid dermal filler injections in photodamaged human skin. Arch Dermatol 2007;143(2):155–63; with permission.)

dermis.[36] The G′ of commonly used HA dermal fillers are included in **Table 1**.

FUTURE USES OF HYALURONIC ACID IN TISSUE ENGINEERING

HA has been studied extensively as a biocompatible, biodegradable, nonimmunogenic material for tissue engineering purposes, including drug delivery, a coating material,[38] for osmotically driven swelling of collagen scaffolds,[32] and as a hydrogel with neurotrophic factors for neural regeneration.[39] In one study, HA was combined with gelatin and seeded with keratinocytes and dermal fibroblasts for skin tissue engineering purposes with the potential of being used for extensive burn victims.[40] Hydrogels composed of HA have been studied for corneal endothelial tissue engineering,[41] as an injectable therapy to prevent left ventricular remodeling following myocardial infarction,[42] as a scaffold for controlled release of dexamethasone for adipose-derived stem cell tissue engineering,[43] and even as a bio-ink for 3-dimensional printing for potential organ fabrication.[44]

ADVERSE EFFECTS

Although adverse effects of HA injectables for soft tissue augmentation are relatively uncommon in the hands of an experienced injector, potential adverse events must be discussed with patients. The most serious complication of HA fillers involves injection into or around the facial vasculature. FDA reports of adverse events associated with HA injections include bruising, erythema, swelling, pain, itching, and, more rarely, infection or abscesses, raised bumps, allergic reactions, or tissue necrosis.[45] Reported adverse effects most commonly include pain at the injection site, swelling, bruising, erythema, small lumps,[19] and development of a postinjection site infection.[6] In one report evaluating Juvéderm in 70 healthy volunteers, one patient developed an abscess at the injection site following prior polyacrylamide injections.[6] Recurrent herpes labialis has been reported following injection of NASHA products.[5]

Injection into or compromise of the local vascular supply due to compression is a rare but potentially devastating complication leading to tissue necrosis and infection.[13,19] Although there is debate as to whether vascular compromise is caused by local compression by the injected filler or embolization or thrombosis from direct injection into a vessel, the treatment remains the same. If there is any sign of vascular compromise such as severe pain, blanching, or tissue duskiness, hyaluronidase and nitropaste should be used

expediently. Skin necrosis following HA injection has been reported in a case report from Iran.[46] All HA gels are clear and may result in a slightly visible blue hue injected too superficially; this may be treated with hyaluronidase. In another case report, 3 patients developed lip nodules 4 to 24 months following Restylane injection.[47] These nodules were excised and found to consist of amorphous hematoxyphilic material surrounded by collagenized connective tissue on histology.[47]

Avoiding anticoagulants, aspirin, and supplements like vitamin E 1 to 2 weeks before injection can reduce postinjection ecchymosis.[13] Patients with a history of herpes infections should take prophylactic valacyclovir for 3 days starting the day before injection.[13] An outstanding knowledge of facial anatomy including precise location of the supraorbital and infraorbital foramen, angular and supratrochlear arteries, are important for safe practice.[33]

SUMMARY

HA injectible fillers are used extensively for soft tissue volumizing and contouring and have increased in popularity over the past 15 years. Many different HA injectable fillers are available on the market and differ in terms of HA concentration, particle size, cross-linking density, requisite needle size, duration, G′, hydration, presence of lidocaine, type of cross-linking technology, and cost. The facial plastic practitioner should be cognizant of these differences for optimal patient outcomes. HA is a natural component of many soft tissues, has been linked to wound healing and skin regeneration, and is currently actively being studied for tissue engineering purposes. Its effect on fibroblast morphology to induce collagen production indirectly (without binding the fibroblasts) as well as its volumizing and osmotic swelling properties lend clear advantages to HA fillers over other types of soft tissue fillers. Knowledge of the tissue device interface and how this affects soft tissue augmentation will help guide the clinical practitioner and lead to optimal outcomes for patients.

REFERENCES

1. 2000/2013/2014 National Cosmetic Procedures. In: plasticsurgery.org. ed: American Society of Plastic Surgeons; 2015. Accessed August 16, 2015.
2. Rydell N, Balazs EA. Effect of intra-articular injection of hyaluronic acid on the clinical symptoms of osteoarthritis and on granulation tissue formation. Clin Orthop Relat Res 1971;80:25–32.

3. Crafoord S, Stenkula S. Healon GV in posterior segment surgery. Acta Ophthalmol (Copenh) 1993; 71(4):560–1.

4. Ghersetich I, Lotti T, Campanile G, et al. Hyaluronic acid in cutaneous intrinsic aging. Int J Dermatol 1994;33(2):119–22.

5. Andre P. Evaluation of the safety of a non-animal stabilized hyaluronic acid (NASHA – Q-Medical, Sweden) in European countries: a retrospective study from 1997 to 2001. J Eur Acad Dermatol Venereol 2004;18(4):422–5.

6. Hoffmann K. Volumizing effects of a smooth, highly cohesive, viscous 20-mg/mL hyaluronic acid volumizing filler: prospective European study. BMC Dermatol 2009;9:9.

7. Caton T, Thibeault SL, Klemuk S, et al. Viscoelasticity of hyaluronan and nonhyaluronan based vocal fold injectables: implications for mucosal versus muscle use. Laryngoscope 2007;117(3):516–21.

8. Baspeyras M, Rouvrais C, Liegard L, et al. Clinical and biometrological efficacy of a hyaluronic acid-based mesotherapy product: a randomised controlled study. Arch Dermatol Res 2013;305(8): 673–82.

9. Medical Device Definition. In: http://www.fda.gov/MedicalDevices/DeviceRegulationandGuidance/Overview/ClassifyYourDevice/ucm051512.htm. ed, Food and Drug Administration. Accessed August 16, 2015.

10. Wang F, Garza LA, Kang S, et al. In vivo stimulation of de novo collagen production caused by cross-linked hyaluronic acid dermal filler injections in photodamaged human skin. Arch Dermatol 2007; 143(2):155–63.

11. Quan T, Wang F, Shao Y, et al. Enhancing structural support of the dermal microenvironment activates fibroblasts, endothelial cells, and keratinocytes in aged human skin in vivo. J Invest Dermatol 2013; 133(3):658–67.

12. Girardeau-Hubert S, Teluob S, Pageon H, et al. The reconstructed skin model as a new tool for investigating in vitro dermal fillers: increased fibroblast activity by hyaluronic acid. Eur J Dermatol 2015. [Epub ahead of print].

13. Baumann L. Dermal fillers. J Cosmet Dermatol 2004; 3(4):249–50.

14. Simoni R, Hill RL, Vaughan M, et al. The discovery of hyaluronan by Karl Meyer. J Biol Chem 2002; 277:e27.

15. Anderegg U, Simon JC, Averbeck M. More than just a filler—the role of hyaluronan for skin homeostasis. Exp Dermatol 2014;23(5):295–303.

16. Cermelli C, Cuoghi A, Scuri M, et al. In vitro evaluation of antiviral and virucidal activity of a high molecular weight hyaluronic acid. Virol J 2011;8:141.

17. Edwards PC, Fantasia JE. Review of long-term adverse effects associated with the use of chemically-modified animal and nonanimal source hyaluronic acid dermal fillers. Clin Interv Aging 2007;2(4):509–19.

18. Gold MH. What's new in fillers in 2010? J Clin Aesthet Dermatol 2010;3(8):36–45.

19. Beasley KL, Weiss MA, Weiss RA. Hyaluronic acid fillers: a comprehensive review. Facial Plast Surg 2009;25(2):86–94.

20. Huss FR, Nyman E, Bolin JS, et al. Use of macroporous gelatine spheres as a biodegradable scaffold for guided tissue regeneration of healthy dermis in humans: an in vivo study. J Plast Reconstr Aesthet Surg 2010;63(5):848–57.

21. Sadick NS, Manhas-Bhutani S, Krueger N. A novel approach to structural facial volume replacement. Aesthet Plast Surg 2013;37(2):266–76.

22. Rohrich RJ, Ghavami A, Crosby MA. The role of hyaluronic acid fillers (Restylane) in facial cosmetic surgery: review and technical considerations. Plast Reconstr Surg 2007;120(Suppl 6):41S–54S.

23. Bogdan Allemann I, Baumann L. Hyaluronic acid gel (Juvederm) preparations in the treatment of facial wrinkles and folds. Clin Interv Aging 2008;3(4): 629–34.

24. Ballin AC, Cazzaniga A, Brandt FS. Long-term efficacy, safety and durability of Juvederm(R) XC. Clin Cosmet Investig Dermatol 2013;6:183–9.

25. Tran C, Carraux P, Micheels P, et al. In vivo biointegration of three hyaluronic acid fillers in human skin: a histological study. Dermatology 2014; 228(1):47–54.

26. Monheit GD, Baumann LS, Gold MH, et al. Novel hyaluronic acid dermal filler: dermal gel extra physical properties and clinical outcomes. Dermatol Surg 2010;36(Suppl 3):1833–41.

27. Gold MH. Use of hyaluronic acid fillers for the treatment of the aging face. Clin Interv Aging 2007;2(3): 369–76.

28. Kim ZH, Lee Y, Kim SM, et al. A composite dermal filler comprising cross-linked hyaluronic acid and human collagen for tissue reconstruction. J Microbiol Biotechnol 2015;25(3):399–406.

29. Richter AW, Ryde EM, Zetterstrom EO. Non-immunogenicity of a purified sodium hyaluronate preparation in man. Int Arch Allergy Appl Immunol 1979; 59(1):45–8.

30. Klein AW, Fagien S. Hyaluronic acid fillers and botulinum toxin type a: rationale for their individual and combined use for injectable facial rejuvenation. Plast Reconstr Surg 2007;120(Suppl 6):81S–8S.

31. Park KY, Ko EJ, Kim BJ, et al. A multicenter, randomized, double-blind clinical study to evaluate the efficacy and safety of PP-501-B in correction of nasolabial folds. Dermatol Surg 2015;41(1): 113–20.

32. Anandagoda N, Ezra DG, Cheema U, et al. Hyaluronan hydration generates three-dimensional

meso-scale structure in engineered collagen tissues. J R Soc Interf 2012;9(75):2680–7.

33. Matarasso SL, Carruthers JD, Jewell ML. Consensus recommendations for soft-tissue augmentation with nonanimal stabilized hyaluronic acid (Restylane). Plast Reconstr Surg 2006;117(Suppl 3):3S–34S [discussion: 35S–43S].

34. Mashiko T, Mori H, Kato H, et al. Semipermanent volumization by an absorbable filler: onlay injection technique to the bone. Plast Reconstr Surg Glob Open 2013;1(1). pii:e4–e14.

35. Fisher GJ, Kang S, Varani J, et al. Mechanisms of photoaging and chronological skin aging. Arch Dermatol 2002;138(11):1462–70.

36. Pierre S, Liew S, Bernardin A. Basics of dermal filler rheology. Dermatol Surg 2015;41(Suppl 1):S120–6.

37. Janmey PA, Georges PC, Hvidt S. Basic rheology for biologists. Methods Cell Biol 2007;83:3–27.

38. Arnal-Pastor M, Valles-Lluch A, Keicher M, et al. Coating typologies and constrained swelling of hyaluronic acid gels within scaffold pores. J Colloid Interf Sci 2011;361(1):361–9.

39. Wei YT, Tian WM, Yu X, et al. Hyaluronic acid hydrogels with IKVAV peptides for tissue repair and axonal regeneration in an injured rat brain. Biomed Mater 2007;2(3):S142–6.

40. Wang TW, Wu HC, Huang YC, et al. Biomimetic bilayered gelatin-chondroitin 6 sulfate-hyaluronic acid biopolymer as a scaffold for skin equivalent tissue engineering. Artif Organs 2006;30(3):141–9.

41. Lai JY, Cheng HY, Ma DH. Investigation of overrun-processed porous hyaluronic acid carriers in corneal endothelial tissue engineering. PLoS One 2015;10(8):e0136067.

42. Dorsey SM, McGarvey JR, Wang H, et al. MRI evaluation of injectable hyaluronic acid-based hydrogel therapy to limit ventricular remodeling after myocardial infarction. Biomaterials 2015;69:65–75.

43. Fan M, Ma Y, Zhang Z, et al. Biodegradable hyaluronic acid hydrogels to control release of dexamethasone through aqueous Diels-Alder chemistry for adipose tissue engineering. Mater Sci Eng C Mater Biol Appl 2015;56:311–7.

44. Shim JH, Kim JY, Park M, et al. Development of a hybrid scaffold with synthetic biomaterials and hydrogel using solid freeform fabrication technology. Biofabrication 2011;3(3):034102.

45. Soft Tissue Fillers (Dermal Fillers). In: http://www.fda.gov/MedicalDevices/ProductsandMedicalProcedures/CosmeticDevices/WrinkleFillers/ucm2007470.htm. ed: U.S. Food and Drug Administration. Accessed August 16, 2015.

46. Manafi A, Barikbin B, Hamedi ZS, et al. Nasal alar necrosis following hyaluronic acid injection into nasolabial folds: a case report. World J Plast Surg 2015;4(1):74–8.

47. Shahrabi Farahani S, Sexton J, Stone JD, et al. Lip nodules caused by hyaluronic acid filler injection: report of three cases. Head Neck Pathol 2012;6(1):16–20.

The Case for Synthetic Injectables

John H. Joseph, MD

KEYWORDS

- Synthetic fillers • Dermal fillers • Permanent fillers • Liquid injectable silicone
- Polymethyl methacrylate • Acne scarring • Nasolabial folds

KEY POINTS

- Bellafill (previously known as Artefill) has been marketed and sold in the United States as a permanent dermal filler for the correction of nasolabial folds since 2007 and received FDA approval for acne scarring in December 2014.
- Bellafill is currently the only "on-label" dermal filler approved by the FDA for the treatment of moderate to severe, atrophic, distensible facial acne scars on the cheeks of patients over the age of 21.
- The number of subjects affected by granuloma in the 5-year Bellafill postmarketing study was small (1.7%), with most events being mild to moderate in severity.
- Liquid injectable silicone was the first highly popularized injectable filler and is one of the oldest and longest lasting.
- Medical-grade silicone oil used off label for soft tissue augmentation with the correct indications and with the microdroplet technique is safe and economic permanent dermal filler.

INTRODUCTION

With the wide acceptance of temporary fillers, such as hyaluronic acid (HA), it is easy to see why permanent fillers with longer-lasting effects are quickly gaining popularity.[1] According to the American Society for Plastic Surgery Procedural Statistics, there were 2.2 million soft tissue filler procedures performed in 2013, representing an increase of 13% over prior year.[2] It is not uncommon for patients who experience superior results with temporary fillers to request more permanent enhancements.[1] Their tolerance for the inconvenience and repeat cost of short-term, temporary fillers is waning as newer-generation fillers with longer durations are coming on the market (Joseph J, Eaton L, Cohen S. Current concepts in the use of Bellafill. Submitted for publication).

Before the modern era of injectable collagen and HA as dermal fillers, several unapproved materials were used. The first permanent facial filler in the twentieth century was paraffin oil.[1] This was followed by a variety of other synthetic fillers, such as mineral oil, linseed oil, beeswax, and lanolin.[1] Medical-grade silicone was approved in 1959 by the US Food and Drug Administration (FDA). Liquid injectable silicone (LIS) oil has been used as permanent soft tissue filler in aesthetics for more than half a century under the auspices of "off-label use of an approved medical device."[1]

There are currently more than 200 dermal fillers and volume enhancers available internationally.[3] In the United States, the Center for Devices and Radiologic Health division of the FDA regulates injectable dermal fillers as medical devices. To receive a premarketing approval in the United States, a medical device manufacturer must demonstrate safety and effectiveness supported by human clinical studies for specific indications, such as "moderate to severe wrinkles and folds."

9400 Brighton Way, Suite 203, Beverly Hills, CA 90210, USA
E-mail address: drjohnjoseph@sbcglobal.net

Facial Plast Surg Clin N Am 23 (2015) 433–445
http://dx.doi.org/10.1016/j.fsc.2015.07.003
1064-7406/15/$ – see front matter © 2015 Elsevier Inc. All rights reserved.

Approval typically requires clinical evidence supported by a US, multicenter, randomized pivotal study using the approved standard of care, which historically was collagen, as a comparator. With more new fillers coming on the US market, head-to-head clinical trials between products of the same or similar type are now the gold standard. Only first-in-class fillers tend to gain approval with a single-arm study, or by using a no-treatment control as a comparator.

Currently there is no universally accepted classification system for injectable fillers; however, the source of the filler may be categorized as natural/animal, synthetic, or natural synthetic.[1] Fillers are further classified by the duration of effect, such as temporary, semipermanent, or permanent.[1] Permanent fillers are basically nonresorbable.[1] This article addresses two products that are currently being used as permanent soft tissue fillers in the United States: polymethyl methacrylate (PMMA) (eg, Bellafill) and LIS oil used in an off-label capacity.

LIQUID INJECTABLE SILICONE
Overview

LIS was the first highly popularized injectable filler and is one of the oldest and longest lasting.[4] LIS is not FDA approved as dermal filler; however, highly purified liquid silicone oil is frequently used "off-label" as a medical device for soft tissue augmentation, such as facial volumizing of lips and cheeks, or as filler for correction of facial wrinkles and folds, such as glabellar lines and nasolabial folds (NLFs). LIS is highly purified long-chain polydimethylsiloxane trimethylsiloxy terminated silicone oil, which is a sterile, generally inert, nonpyrogenic, clear, colorless oil with a viscosity of 1000 centistokes.[5,6] Silicone oil is well accepted because of its natural feel and ease of injection,[1] and is well tolerated in small volumes.[1,7–10] The mechanism of action of silicone oil is the stimulation of a fibrotic reaction within the dermis, which is followed by low-grade inflammation and subsequent capsule formation.[1]

Legal Status of Liquid Injectable Silicone

FDA guidance on "off-label" use of marketed drug and devices allows for physicians to use legally available products for an indication that is not in the approved labeling, providing that the physician uses good medical practice in the best interest of the patient, is well informed about the product, bases its use on firm scientific rationale and on sound medical evidence, and maintains records of the product's use and effects.[11]

Product Information

Two forms of LIS are FDA approved as medical devices in the United State, both for use in ophthalmology as retinal stabilizing agents. Silikon 1000 (Alcon, Ft. Worth, TX) is available in 10-mL glass vials filled with 8.5 mL of sterile silicone oil,[5] and ADATO Sil-Ol-5000 silicone oil (Bausch + Lomb, Rochester, NY) is available in prefilled syringes. Silicone oil is found in abundance from manufacturers in Mexico and South America; however, these formulations may contain impurities that can results in undesirable complications.[1] Therefore, their use should be strictly avoided.

Patient Selection

Any facial defect can be examined for filling with silicone, including thin lips, nasal defects, smoker's lines, glabellar frown lines, NLFs, poorly defined cheekbones or chins, or postsurgical deformities. Broad-based facial scars from trauma or surgery (**Figs. 1** and **2**), and acne scars that disappear with manual stretching, are good candidates for treatment with silicone. Patients who are pregnant, are nursing, or who have active skin infections or uncontrolled systemic diseases are not candidates.

Silicone Injection: Microdroplet Technique

The ideal injection technique of silicone oil as a facial filler, after the treatment area has been cleaned and prepared, consists of microdroplet application with a 27-gauge by 0.5-inch needle, or with a 25- or 27-gauge microcannula into the dermal-subcutaneous junction.[7–9,12] After entering the skin at a 30° angle, fluid silicone is injected in a retrograde fashion at 2- to 4-mm intervals,[4,13] starting outside of the perimeter of the depressed area. For larger areas, multiple passes with a fanning injection technique may be required. Serial puncture technique of 0.05- to 0.1-mL aliquots of LIS is also a commonly used way to administrator the microdroplets of LIS in the area to be treated. Multiple treatment sessions are usually required to obtain the desired outcome. The microdroplet injection technique requires spacing the injections by at least a month or longer to allow adequate fibroplasia to occur.[13] The injected microdroplets of silicone become surrounded by a capsule of collagenous fibrous tissue, which holds them in place and minimizes migration.[13] In addition, this gradual fibroplasia ensures the injected area has the same texture as the adjacent tissue and that the product is not palpable.[13]

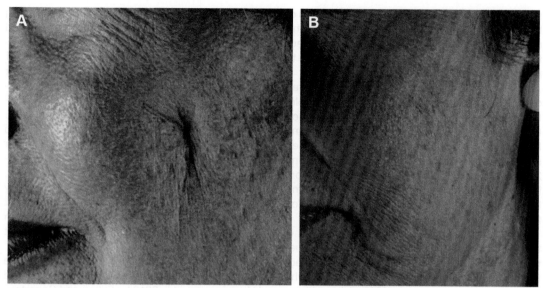

Fig. 1. (A) Baseline photograph of female patient with facial scarring to left cheek to be treated with liquid injectable silicone. (B) Posttreatment of scar on left cheek that was treated with liquid injectable silicone. (Courtesy of D.M. Duffy, MD, Torrance, CA.)

The Case for Liquid Silicone: Clinical Data Supporting its Use for Facial Soft Tissue Augmentation

An abundance of published literature, dating back almost 40 years, provides clinical evidence that purified medical-grade silicone oil, when used judiciously by experienced clinicians for facial soft tissue augmentation, can provide safe and effective outcomes. In 1986 Webster and colleagues[8] reported on 20 years of experience using LIS in postrhinoplasty patients. Three hundred forty-seven patients were treated with a total of 1937 treatments.[8] The product was used conservatively with cautious injection of small amounts of silicone using the microdroplet technique. This

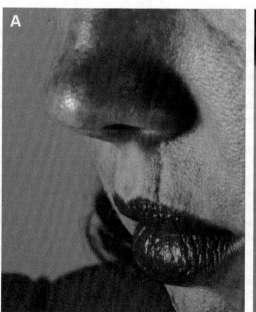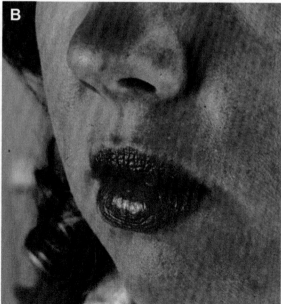

Fig. 2. (A) Female patient with scar above lip, planned for treatment with liquid injectable silicone. (B) Posttreatment of scarring above the lip treated with liquid injectable silicone. (Courtesy of D.M. Duffy, MD, Torrance, CA.)

study demonstrated that using very small doses of LIS is a safe and effective adjunct to cosmetic rhinoplastic procedures and can be used for correction of nasal defects that may not be amenable to revisional surgery.[8]

Also, in 1986 Webster and colleagues[9] reported on a 20-year experience using the microdroplet technique for liquid silicone injection performed for camouflaging furrows and groves, augmenting facial eminences, and elevating certain depressed scars. The report spanned 235 patients, including 2811 treatments. This study supported other work indicating induction of collagen deposition around the microdroplets, thus providing augmentation from volumes of collagen and silicone.[9]

Hevia[14] reported on his 6-year experience in treating patients with 1000-centistoke polydimethylsiloxane in his private practice. This retrospective chart review included 916 patients who received 5246 treatments in 3307 visits, with an average of 3.5 visits per patients and 1.6 treatments per visit.[14] Treatment areas included facial rhytides, acne scars, lips, infraorbital, nasolabial, and general contours. Adverse events were limited to overcorrection in 11 patients (1%).[14] This study concluded that PDSM-1000 was found to be effective and safe in the cosmetic practice setting.[14]

Duffy[10] reported on his 22-year experience involving the treatment of more than 3000 patients using LIS and concluded that pure silicone may be superior to any currently available agent in properly selected patients for permanent correction of certain types of defects. Jones and colleagues[12] reported data on 77 patients suffering from human immunodeficiency virus–associated lipoatrophy who were treated with LIS. In this study, supple and even facial contours were routinely restored, all patients tolerated the treatments well, and no adverse events were noted.[12]

In 2010, Moscona and Fodor[15] published the results of a 179 patient retrospective study of LIS for lip augmentation. The microdroplet technique was used in all cases, and not more than 1 mL per lip per session was injected. Long-term results (3–7 years), satisfaction level, and complications were evaluated. Eighty-five percent of the patients reported excellent or good results. Most (76%) patients considered their lips to be as soft as they were before treatment. No complications were recorded for 91.1% of the patients. Complications encountered by the rest were minor and temporary, such as ecchymosis and hematoma in 6.2%, and invisible but small palpable nodules in 2.2%. This study concluded that LIS is safe for a period of 3 to 7 years and gives a high level of patient satisfaction with minimal complications.[15]

A 10-year experience across 206 cases using LIS for soft tissue augmentation was conducted by Jacinto[16] in the Philippines. Most (82%) patients were female and between the ages of 21 and 30 years. Fifty-five percent were treated for acne scars, 42% nasolabial grooves, 13.5% marionette lines, 12.6% glabellar lines, 9.8% postvaricella scars, 9.3% inframalar depressions, 1.8% posttraumatic scars, 1.4% lipodystrophy, 1% lip augmentation, 0.9% sleep lines, and 0.4% contour defects. Seventy-two percent had excellent results, 18% had good results, 2% had fair results, and only 0.5% had poor results. This study concluded that silicone oil injected with the correct indications and with the microdroplet injection technique is a safe, economical, and permanent dermal and subcutaneous filler.[16]

A simple yet permanent method of tissue augmentation using an emulsification of LIS and HA was reported in 2012 by Fulton and Caperton[4] (N = 95) in which they mixed 0.5 mL of 1000 centistoke LIS with 1 mL of cross-linked HA, such as Restylane or Juvederm, into an emulsion between two 3-mL Luer-lock syringes connected with a Luer-lock to Luer-lock adapter. The emulsion was then injected through either a 27-gauge needle or through a 25- or 27-gauge microcannula into the mid-dermis, subcutaneous tissue, or periosteum. They found the emulsion provided immediate improvement in depressions, folds, and facial contours. It was most beneficial for distensible acne valleys; NLFs; glabellar frown lines; augmentation of the vermillion border of the lips; and projection of the nose, cheekbones, and chin. Exterior nasal deviations and soft tissue defects were also improved. Complications were minimal and included temporary bruising, erythema, and mild edema. Small, temporary nodules were easily leveled with massage and no cases developed silicone granuloma. This study found that treatment remained stable during the 2-year follow-up period.[4]

Histologic evidence

Zappi and colleagues[17] performed 35 skin biopsies, which were examined by light microscopy on 25 patients who had been injected with liquid silicone for soft tissue augmentation procedures between 1 and 23 years prior. The microscopic study revealed in 100% of the cases the continued presence, in significant amounts, of the silicone previously injected into the target areas, where it failed to elicit any significant adverse reactions. This study concluded that silicone, because of its high performance and its inertness, reflected by the lack of any adverse reactions to its presence in the target site, should be regarded as valuable filler, at least for the correction of small depressed facial scars.

Complications of Liquid Injectable Silicone

Complications of LIS range from minor to serious. Minor complications include erythema, ecchymosis, and edema that occur at the injection site,[4] which are not specific to LIS and are seen with other fillers.[13]

Injectable silicone, especially of questionable or adulterated sources, has led to some undesirable local and systemic effects. Although considered biologically inert,[13,18] this material has been implicated in a variety of adverse reactions, including reports of chronic cellulitis,[19] inflammatory nodules,[18–21] lesions,[22] migration,[19,21] ulceration,[19] and silicone granuloma formation.[13,18,21,23] Often these complications are the result of the use of industrial grade silicone, which contains many contaminants, injected by unlicensed or unskilled practitioners.[13,18]

All dermal fillers have the potential to cause complications.[24,25] Unintended reactions such as granulomas, infections, and vascular occlusion, can follow treatment with LIS.[6] Injecting physicians must be aware of these potential complications because early medical care and treatment may help minimize the consequences for the patient and the physician.

Silicone Discussion

LIS has many individual characteristics that physicians would classify as "ideal" for a soft tissue augmentation agent.[13] It is odorless, colorless, nonvolatile, noncarcinogenic, thermally stable to allow heat sterilization, chemically stable when stored at room temperature for long periods of time, and does not have to be reconstituted before use.[13]

Over the years, the use of LIS for soft tissue augmentation has been associated with a great deal of controversy and negative publicity. Although historical complications have occurred, likely resulting from the presence of adulterants and impurities, modern purified silicone products approved by the FDA for injection into the human body may be used with minimal complications when strict protocol is followed.[26] Although its use remains controversial, LIS is an important and effective dermal filler for long-term correction of scarring and facial contour defects.

Although the quality of the product has significantly improved, in terms of purity, several severe adverse events have been published,[27] and the product remains off-label in the United States. The treatment time is limited, the patient discomfort and morbidity are minimal, and the results are long lasting[7]; however, physicians must be advised that the misuse of this agent or other materials masquerading as medical-grade LIS have created a pervasive climate of distrust and a veritable minefield of negative medicolegal possibilities.[10]

Medical-grade silicone oil used off label for soft tissue augmentation, with the correct indications and with the microdroplet injection technique, is a safe and economical permanent dermal filler. Rare permanent erythematous papules and transient ecchymosis appear on deep dermal injections.[16] Unfortunately, no large-scale and randomized FDA clinical trials have been conducted seeking FDA approval for an aesthetic indication for LIS; therefore the jury is still out on its confirmed safety and effectiveness for soft tissue augmentation. Despite this fact, LIS has still been used successfully in facial aesthetics for more than half a century.

POLYMETHYL METHACRYLATE
Overview

PMMA was first used as a biocompatible cement in neurosurgery, joint replacement, and otolaryngology.[28] The proposed mechanism of action for PMMA microspheres is that they impart volume restoration by providing scaffolding that promotes neocollagenesis.[29]

Product Information

Bellafill (Suneva Medical, San Diego, CA) is a long-lasting PMMA injectable filler.[30] It is nonbiodegradeable and composed of 30- to 50-μm smooth and round PMMA microspheres (20% by volume) suspended in a water-based gel containing 3.5% bovine collagen (80% by volume) and 0.3% lidocaine.[29] Although the collagen carrier is absorbed 1 to 3 months after injection, the PMMA microspheres remain as a scaffold for the development of autologous tissue.[29] The bovine collagen carrier is replaced by the patient's own connective tissue over an estimated period of 3 months.[29]

Bellafill (previously known as Artefill) has been marketed and sold in the United States as a permanent dermal filler for the correction of NLFs since 2007 (**Figs. 3** and **4**) and received FDA approval for acne scarring in December 2014 (**Figs. 5–7**). With this new indication, Bellafill is currently the only "on-label" dermal filler approved by the FDA for the treatment of moderate to severe, atrophic, distensible facial acne scars on the cheeks of patients older than the age of 21 (Joseph J, Eaton L, Cohen S. Current concepts in the use of Bellafill. Submitted for publication).

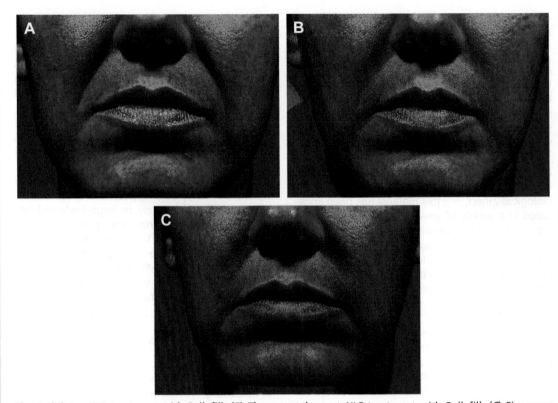

Fig. 3. (*A*) Pre–NLF treatment with Bellafill. (*B*) Three months post–NLF treatment with Bellafill. (*C*) Five years post–NLF treatment with Bellafill.

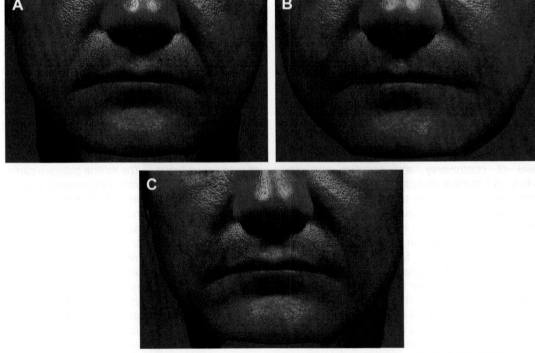

Fig. 4. (*A*) Pre–NLF treatment with Bellafill. (*B*) Three months post–NLF treatment with Bellafill. (*C*) Five years post–NLF treatment with Bellafill.

Before

12 Months

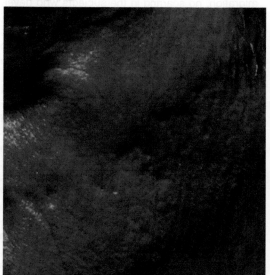

Fig. 5. Baseline and 12 months post–acne scar treatment with Bellafill. Only select scars were treated, not the entire cheek.

The Case for Polymethyl Methacrylate (Bellafill)

Bellafill 5-year postmarketing nasolabial fold study

A concern for the use of permanent, synthetic dermal fillers is the safety profile of long-lasting product. Some clinicians have specifically avoided the use of these fillers for fear of this complication; however, the information they have used to base decisions surrounding PMMA has primarily come from small single-center studies, or case reports in which the precise material administered was not clearly identified, or even FDA approved.[31]

As a condition of the original premarketing approval of Bellafill for NLFs, the FDA required the manufacturer (Suneva Medical, Inc) to conduct

Before

12 Months

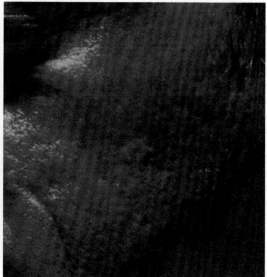

Fig. 6. Baseline and 12 months post–acne scar treatment with Bellafill. Only select scars were treated, not the entire cheek.

Before

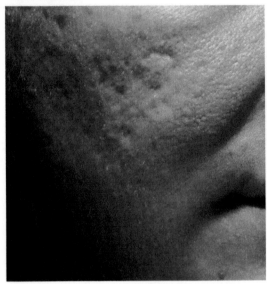

12 Months

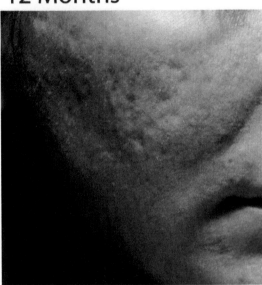

Fig. 7. Baseline and 12 months post–acne scar treatment with Bellafill. Only select scars were treated, not the entire cheek.

a large-scale, 5-year postmarketing study on the safety and satisfaction of long-term treatment (Joseph J, Eaton L, Cohen S. Current concepts in the use of Bellafill. Submitted for publication). As requested by the agency, a prospective, multicenter, open-label postapproval NLF study was conducted at 23 centers across the United States. A total of 1217 subjects were screened and 1008 were enrolled. Compliance with follow-up was outstanding, with 87% completers (871 of 1008) at 5 years (Joseph J, Eaton L, Cohen S. Current concepts in the use of Bellafill. Submitted for publication).

A total of 177 treatment-related adverse events (TRAEs) were reported in 118 of the 1008 Bellafill-treated subjects. Most (74%) TRAEs were mild in severity and resolved within 180 days. The most commonly reported adverse events were lumpiness at the injection site (29%) and redness (10%) (Joseph J, Eaton L, Cohen S. Current concepts in the use of Bellafill. Submitted for publication). Seventeen subjects presented with lesions that were classified, per protocol and biopsy, as granulomas, for an overall incidence rate of 1.7%. Most confirmed granulomas were mild to moderate in severity. Of the 17 subjects with granuloma, eight had complete resolution, eight were improving with ongoing treatment at the end of the study, and one granuloma initially improved and then remained stable for the last two study visits. Of the lesions that resolved, the average duration was 10 months (range, 2.5–21 months) (Joseph J, Eaton L, Cohen S. Current

concepts in the use of Bellafill. Submitted for publication).

Subjects with granulomas were treated with a variety of medical treatment modalities. The most commonly used treatment was intralesional corticosteroid injections with and without intralesional 5-fluorouracil. No implants were excised or removed (Joseph J, Eaton L, Cohen S. Current concepts in the use of Bellafill. Submitted for publication). Additionally, there were no reports of migration, no scarring in the subjects who developed granulomas, no blindness, no infarction, and no symptoms of vascular compromise in this 5-year study of more than 1000 patients (Joseph J, Eaton L, Cohen S. Current concepts in the use of Bellafill. Submitted for publication).

This study represents the largest and longest follow-up study of a US-approved dermal filler product to date and clearly defines the risk of granuloma formation with PMMA-collagen (Joseph J, Eaton L, Cohen S. Current concepts in the use of Bellafill. Submitted for publication). The number of subjects affected by granuloma in the 5-year Bellafill postmarketing study was small (1.7%), with most events being mild to moderate in severity and treatable with medical therapy (Joseph J, Eaton L, Cohen S. Current concepts in the use of Bellafill. Submitted for publication). Although the short-term safety of Bellafill was already well known, this larger long-term study further confirms the overall mild and transient nature of adverse events that can occur with

PMMA-collagen (Joseph J, Eaton L, Cohen S. Current concepts in the use of Bellafill. Submitted for publication).

Bellafill US Acne Scar pivotal study

The Bellafill US Acne Scar pivotal study was a prospective, randomized, placebo-controlled, multicenter, double-blinded clinical trial of subjects older than the age of 18 who desired correction of moderate to severe, atrophic, distensible facial acne scarring on the cheek. The study treated 147 subjects at 10 centers. Subjects who met all inclusion criteria and no exclusion criteria were randomized in a 2:1 fashion to either Bellafill or sterile normal saline solution for injection (Control group). At 6 months, all control subjects were eligible to receive open-label treatment with Bellafill (Joseph J, Eaton L, Cohen S. Current concepts in the use of Bellafill. Submitted for publication).

The primary effectiveness end point was the success rate at 6 months based on the blinded Evaluating Investigator's (EI) assessment using Suneva's validated four-point Acne Scar Rating Scale (ASRS) with success defined as at least a two-point improvement on the ASRS for at least 50% of treated scars, and the primary safety objective was to identify the incidence of all adverse events (Joseph J, Eaton L, Cohen S. Current concepts in the use of Bellafill. Submitted for publication).

The study enrolled male and female subjects, 18 years of age or older, who presented with at least four moderate to severe atrophic acne scars on the cheeks that were sufficiently distant from one another to allow for individual treatment and grading. Treatment scars had to be depressed rolling scars with rounded borders, distensible, and not significantly hypopigmented or hyperpigmented, with no underlying papules or nodules. Icepick, boxcar, or bound-down acne scars could not be included as treatable scars, but could be present in the treatment area.

Exclusion criteria included a recent or current history of inflammatory skin disease; infection; cancerous/precancerous lesions; unhealed wounds; or clinically significant acne, which was defined as greater than three active inflammatory lesions in either the left or right treatment area. Other study exclusion criteria included a history of systemic granulomatous diseases; connective tissue disorders; hypertrophic acne scarring; keloid scarring; predominantly icepick scarring or sinus tract scars; and a known hypersensitivity or previous allergic reaction to any of the components Bellafill, including lidocaine and bovine collagen. Additional inclusion and exclusion criteria were outlined in the study protocol.

End points measured after treatment included (1) the masked EIs determination of acne scar severity via the four-point validated ASRS, (2) assessment of safety outcomes at each visit, (3) the masked EIs assessment of subject improvement using the Global Aesthetic Improvement Scale, (4) the subject's completion of a 14-day treatment diary, (5) the subject's evaluation of improvement using the Global Aesthetic Improvement Scale, and (6) the subject's assessment of scar correction.

The Bellafill and control groups were well balanced with regard to demographics and baseline characteristics with no significant differences between groups. The mean age was 44.6 years in the Bellafill group and 45.3 years in the control group. The study enrolled a substantial portion of males, which included 38.1% in the Bellafill group and 40.0% in the control group, and subjects with Fitzpatrick skin photo types V and VI, with 25.7% in the Bellafill group and 20.0% in the control group. The mean number of qualified/treated scars in the Bellafill group was 8.9 scars and in the control group it was 8.5 scars. The mean severity score of scars was 3.3 in the Bellafill and 3.3 in the control group as per the ASRS.

The average initial injection volume of Bellafill was 0.11 mL per scar, and the average initial volume injected per subject was 0.93 mL. The average injection volume at touch-up was 0.10 mL per scar and 0.69 mL per subject. Most subjects received a touch-up injection with 82.5% in the Bellafill group and 82.0% in the control group.

The primary effectiveness end point was defined as a responder rate analysis at 6 months in which the criterion for success was greater than or equal to 50% of treated scars (per subject) was improved by two or more points on the four-point ASRS, as evaluated by a masked live EI. The primary effectiveness end point was achieved with 64.4% responders in the Bellafill group and 32.6% responders in the control group (P = .0005).[32] (Joseph J, Eaton L, Cohen S. Current concepts in the use of Bellafill. Submitted for publication.)

There were no deaths, device-related serious adverse events, infections, or vascular occlusions reported in the Acne Scar pivotal study (Joseph J, Eaton L, Cohen S. Current concepts in the use of Bellafill. Submitted for publication). Subject diary card-reported signs and symptoms included erythema, swelling, bruising, pain, itching, lumps/bumps, and skin discoloration. Eighty-nine percent of subjects reported at least one of these signs or symptoms; however, most events were mild to moderate in intensity and resolved within 1 to 7 days. Investigator-reported TRAEs included implant site mass, injection site pain, injection site reaction (eg, lumpiness and papule formation), swelling, and one case of acne (Joseph J, Eaton L, Cohen S. Current concepts in the use of Bellafill. Submitted for publication). These events occurred in 8 out of 97 subjects who were randomized to receive Bellafill. Five of these events resolved and three cases of injection site reaction (lumpiness and papule formation directly after injection) persisted throughout the study (Joseph J, Eaton L, Cohen S. Current concepts in the use of Bellafill. Submitted for publication).

Adverse events of special interest were followed separately for the study. These included hyperpigmentation and hypopigmentation, hypertrophic scarring or keloid formation, and the appearance of granulomas. None of these adverse events were reported in this 12-month pivotal study (Joseph J, Eaton L, Cohen S. Current concepts in the use of Bellafill. Submitted for publication).

Most (at least 83%) of Bellafill-treated subjects judged themselves to be satisfied with the appearance of their treated scars at all time points. From 3 months onward, greater than 77% of Bellafill-treated subjects indicated that their appearance was improved or much improved (Joseph J, Eaton L, Cohen S. Current concepts in the use of Bellafill. Submitted for publication).

This study was considered a success, in that the 6-month primary effectiveness results demonstrated statistically significant effectiveness (vs placebo control) in the treatment of atrophic acne scarring of the face while maintaining an excellent safety profile.[32] (Joseph J, Eaton L, Cohen S. Current concepts in the use of Bellafill. Submitted for publication.) Most subjects and physicians saw an improvement in the appearance of acne scars when treated with Bellafill at 6 months.[32] Unblinded evaluation out to 12 months confirmed a consistent level of effectiveness (Joseph J, Eaton L, Cohen S. Current concepts in the use of Bellafill. Submitted for publication). This study demonstrates that acne scar treatment with Bellafill occurs quickly and is reliably produced in all genders and ages.[32]

Treatment of Atrophic Acne Scarring with Bellafill

Patient selection and consultation

Patients selected for acne scar treatment with Bellafill should present with atrophic (pitted) distensible scarring on the cheeks. The best results with Bellafill are achieved in distensible defects with full correction being achieved gradually over time (Joseph J, Eaton L, Cohen S. Current concepts in the use of Bellafill. Submitted for

publication). The rate and degree of correction in the implanted area varies with the patient, treatment site, and plane of injection. The key to success with Bellafill is a conservative approach with avoidance of overcorrection.[33] Final correction should be limited to no more than 100% of the skin defect during treatment. One or two touch-up treatments at intervals of at least 2 to 4 weeks may be required to achieve the desired effect.

During the initial patient consultation, using a hand-held mirror, have the patient point out the scars that bother him or her the most. Review the degree of acne scar correction that can be achieved with Bellafill and explain that it may take a series of injections of to obtain optimal correction. Examine the skin of the cheek to ensure that the patient has distensible acne scars (scars that smooth out when stretched), because these rolling, broad-based scars respond best to treatment.[32] (Joseph J, Eaton L, Cohen S. Current concepts in the use of Bellafill. Submitted for publication.) The patient's acne scar contour deficiencies should also be well characterized with regard to cause, distensability, and depth of lesions.

Skin testing and photography

Because of the presence of bovine collagen in the carrier gel, there is a risk of a hypersensitive reaction to the formulation; therefore, Bellafill requires a skin test to be performed 4 weeks before treatment.[29,34] The skin test dose of 0.1 mL of Bellafill should be injected in the volar aspect of the forearm and the patient should be provided with the skin test card to take home and complete.[35] A positive skin test response includes symptoms of erythema, induration, and/or swelling appearing within the first 24 hours and lasting greater than 24 hours after injection, or appearing at any time greater than 24 hours after injection.[35] An equivocal response is one in which there are no local signs or symptoms of skin reaction, but there are systemic signs and symptoms of arthralgias or myalgias.[35] A patient with a positive response or two equivocal responses should not be treated with Bellafill.[35]

Pretreatment and posttreatment photographs are highly recommended, because photographs can be an effective tool to demonstrate the results of acne scar treatment. The appearance of acne scars change with the angles of light and are less apparent in flat light; therefore it is important to position the light source tangential to the surface of the area of skin to be photographed. This creates shallow contours and produces long shadows that highlight scars.[36]

Bellafill injection procedure and technique

Bellafill is designed to be injected into the deep dermis, or right at the dermal/subcutaneous junction. Before injection the patient should be fully informed of the indications, contraindications, warnings, precautions, treatment responses, adverse reactions, and method of administration of Bellafill. Confirm the negative skin test.[35] The treatment area should be thoroughly washed and the area cleaned with an antiseptic. The Bellafill syringe must be brought to room temperature before injection. Each Bellafill syringe comes supplied with a 26-gauge by five-eighths-inch needle.[34]

Acne scar treatment Enter the skin at a 30° angle proximal to the edge of the scar. Advance the needle under the base of the scar and explore for any fibrotic tissue. If scar fibrosis exists then pass the needle back and forth a few times to open up a pocket for injecting the product. You can use either a linear threading or serial puncture technique directly underneath the scar, in both cases injecting in a retrograde fashion. You may need to replace the needle if it becomes occluded or dull during the treatment session. After injection, palpate and massage the injected acne scar with your fingertips to confirm uniform deposition of Bellafill.

Polymethyl Methacrylate Discussion

Bellafill has proved to be safe and well tolerated with excellent posttreatment outcomes.[32] (Joseph J, Eaton L, Cohen S. Current concepts in the use of Bellafill. Submitted for publication.) There were no events of granuloma present in the US Acne Scar pivotal trial, and only a 1.7% incidence of granuloma formation seen in a long-term, 5-year, postapproval study of more than 1000 patients treated with PMMA-collagen for correction of NLF (Joseph J, Eaton L, Cohen S. Current concepts in the use of Bellafill. Submitted for publication).

SUMMARY

For the longest time physicians have avoided the use of permanent fillers for several reasons. First, silicone was initially injected in large boluses in one or two sessions, which resulted in migration of the product to undesirable locations.[37] Clinicians tried to eliminate this problem by adding inflammatory agents to "hold the product in place." This created horrific complications, especially in the breast, and as a result the aesthetic use of silicone was banned in the state of Nevada.[37] These disasters created urban myths surrounding permanent fillers, such as "permanent filler, permanent problem" or terms like "granuloma factory." Second, initial attempts using primitive forms of PMMA and other materials only reinforced these conclusions. However, if one looks carefully at the history and evolution of medical-grade LIS and PMMA (Bellafill) the safety and efficacy of these permanent synthetic fillers is now supported by a mountain of scientific evidence that should no

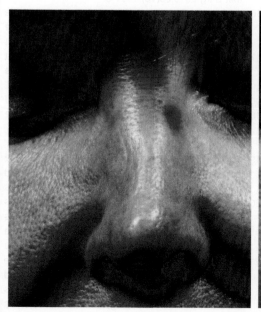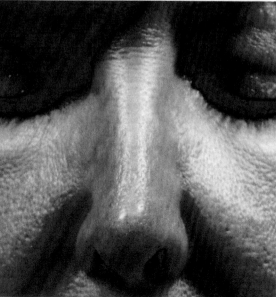

Fig. 8. Baseline and 5-year status postrepair of nasal defect with a permanent synthetic injectable filler.

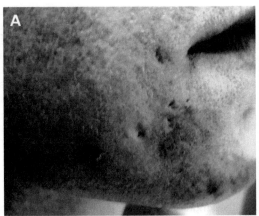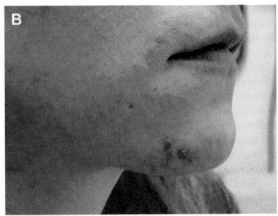

Fig. 9. (*A*) Pre–acne scar treatment with a permanent synthetic injectable filler. (*B*) Post–acne scar treatment with a permanent synthetic injectable filler.

longer be ignored. Permanent synthetic fillers can be used safely and effectively in several areas, including repair of nasal defects (**Fig. 8**), acne scarring (**Fig. 9**), filling of wrinkles and folds, and many other off-label applications.

REFERENCES

1. Wilson Y, Ellis D. Permanent soft tissue fillers. Facial Plast Surg 2011;27(6):540–6.
2. ASPS. ASPS National Clearinghouse of Plastic Surgery Procedural Statistics. Plastic Surgery Statistics Report. 2013. Available at: http://www.plasticsurgery.org/news/plastic-surgery-statistics/2013. Accessed February 25, 2015.
3. Glogau R. Fillers: from the past to the future. Semin Cutan Med Surg 2012;31:78–87.
4. Fulton J, Caperton C. The optimal filler: immediate and long-term results with emulsified silicone (1,000 centistokes) with cross-linked hyaluronic acid. J Drugs Dermatol 2012;11(11):1336–41.
5. Alcon. [Package insert]. Silikon 1000. Ft. Worth, TX: 2013.
6. Hexsel S, de Morais M. Management of complications of injectable silicone. Facial Plast Surg 2014; 30(6):623–7.
7. Orentreich D, Leone A. A case of HIV-associated facial lipoatrophy treated with 1000-cs liquid injectable silicone. Dermatol Surg 2004;30(4 Pt 1): 548–51.
8. Webster R, Hamdan U, Gaunt J, et al. Rhinoplastic revisions with liquid silicone. Arch Otolaryngol Head Neck Surg 1986;112(3):269–76.
9. Webster R, Gaunt J, Hamdan U, et al. Injectable silicone for facial soft-tissue augmentation. Arch Otolaryngol Head Neck Surg 1986;112(3):290–6.
10. Duffy D. Liquid silicone for soft tissue augmentation. Dermatol Surg 2005;31(11 Pt 2):1530–41.
11. FDA. "Off-Label" and investigational use of marketed drugs, biologics, and medical devices: information sheet. 2014.
12. Jones D, Carruthers A, Orentreich D, et al. Highly purified 1000-cSt silicone oil for treatment of human immunodeficiency virus-associated facial lipoatrophy: an open pilot trial. Dermatol Surg 2004;30(10):1279–86.
13. Ellis L, Cohen J, High W. Granulomatous reaction to silicone injection. J Clin Aesthet Dermatol 2012;5(7):44–7.
14. Hevia O. Six-year experience using 1,000-centistoke silicone oil in 916 patients for soft-tissue augmentation in a private practice setting. Dermatol Surg 2009;25(Suppl 2):1646–52.
15. Moscona R, Fodor L. A retrospective study on liquid injectable silicone for lip augmentation: long-term results and patient satisfaction. J Plast Reconstr Aesthet Surg 2010;63(10):1694–8.
16. Jacinto S. Ten-year experience using injectable silicone oil for soft tissue augmentation in the Philippines. Dermatol Surg 2005;31(11 Pt 2):1550–4.
17. Zappi E, Barnett J, Zappi M, et al. The long-term host response to liquid silicone injected during soft tissue augmentation procedures: a microscopic appraisal. Dermatol Surg 2007;33(Suppl 2):S186–92.
18. Schwartzfarb E, Hametti J, Romanelli P, et al. Foreign body granuloma formation secondary to silicone injection. Dermatol Online J 2008;14(7):20.
19. Rapaport M, Vinnik C, Zarem H. Injectable silicone: cause of facial nodules, cellulitis, ulceration, and migration. Aesthetic Plast Surg 1996;20(3):267–76.
20. Ledon J, Savas J, Yang S, et al. Inflammatory nodules following soft tissue filler use: a review of causative agents, pathology, and treatment options. Am J Clin Dermatol 2013;14(5):401–11.
21. Beer K. Delayed onset nodules from liquid injectable silicone: report of a case, evaluation of associated histopathology and results of treatment with minocycline and celocoxib. J Drugs Dermatol 2009;8(10): 952–4.

22. Achauer B. A serious complication following medical-grade silicone injection of the face. Plast Reconstr Surg 1983;71(2):251–4.

23. Anastassov G, Schulhof S, Lumerman H. Complications after facial contour augmentation with injectable silicone. Diagnosis and treatment. Report of a severe case. Int J Oral Maxillofac Surg 2008;37(10):955–60.

24. Funt D, Pavicic T. Dermal fillers in aesthetics: an overview of adverse events and treatment approaches. Plast Surg Nurs 2015;35(1):13–32.

25. DeLorenzi C. Complications of injectable fillers, part 2: vascular complications. Aesthet Surg J 2014;34(4):584–600.

26. Prather C, Jones D. Liquid injectable silicone for soft tissue augmentation. Dermatol Ther 2006;19(3):159–68.

27. Requena C, Izquierdo M, Navarro M, et al. Adverse reactions to injectable aesthetic microimplants. Am J Dermatopathol 2001;23(3):197–202.

28. Cohen S, Berner C, Mariono B, et al. Five-year safety and efficacy of a novel polymethyl-methacrylate aesthetic soft tissue filler for the correction of nasolabial folds. Dermatol Surg 2007;33(Suppl 2):S222–30.

29. Lemperle G, Knapp T, Sadick N, et al. ArteFill Permanent injectable for soft tissue augmentation: I. mechanism of action and injection techniques. Aesthetic Plast Surg 2010;34(3):287–9.

30. Rose AE. Therapeutic update on acne scarring. J Drugs Dermatol 2014;13(6):651–4.

31. Piacquadio D, Smith S, Anderson R. A comparison of commercially available polymethylmethacrylate-based soft tissue fillers. Dermatol Surg 2008;34(Suppl 1):S48–52.

32. Karnik J, Baumann L, Bruce S, et al. A double-blind, randomized, multicenter, controlled trial of suspended polymethylmethcrylate microspheres for the correction of atrophic facial acne scars. J Am Acad Dermatol 2014;71(1):77–83.

33. Hilinski J, Cohen S. Soft tissue augmentation with ArteFill. Facial Plast Surg 2009;25(2):114–9.

34. Suneva. Bellafill instructions for use. 2014.

35. Suneva. Bellafill skin test instructions for use. 2014.

36. Suneva. Suneva before and after photo taking guide. 2014.

37. Duffy D. The silicone conundrum: a battle of anecdotes. Dermatol Surg 2002;28(7):590–5.

Facial Filler Complications

Julie Woodward, MD[a],[*], Tanya Khan, MD[a], John Martin, MD[b]

KEYWORDS

- Facial fillers • Hyaluronic acid • Hyaluronidase • Complications • Granulomas • Biofilms • Necrosis
- Blindness

KEY POINTS

- Identification of various filler-associated adverse events.
- Knowledge of tips to prevent filler-associated adverse events.
- Recognition of vascular occlusions: how to avoid them and how to treat them.

INTRODUCTION

Facial filler injections represent an ever-expanding market of nonsurgical facial rejuvenation. Second only to botulinum toxin type A injections, soft tissue fillers comprised 2.3 million procedures performed in the United States in 2014, a 4.5% increase from the previous year.[1] Approximately 78% (1.8 million) of these 2.3 million total dermal filler injections represent hyaluronic acid (HA) fillers. This specific popularity may be caused by the potential reversibility of the HA fillers with hyaluronidase, which allows injectors and patients the ease of dissolving unwanted filler.

Currently in the United States, the following substances have been Food and Drug Administration (FDA)-approved for treating facial rhytids: autologous fat, collagen (Evolence, Cosmoderm, Fibrel, Zyplast, Zyderm), HA (Restylane-L, Restylane Silk, Juvederm XC, Juvederm Voluma XC, Belotero Balance, Prevelle Silk, Elevess, Captique, Hylaform), poly-(L)-lactic acid (PLLA; Sculptra and Sculptra Aesthetic), calcium hydroxylapatite (Radiesse), and polymethyl methacrylate (PMMA; Bellafill, formerly known as Artefill).[2,3]

Although HA fillers have been touted to be safer and thus more widespread than the other filler types, all have been associated with adverse outcomes. These complications range from localized bruising, erythema, edema, migration, allergic response, the formation of small bumps underneath the skin, to more serious sequelae, such as permanent visual loss and nerve paralysis. Although not approved for domestic use, polyacrylamide gel and other non-FDA-approved substances are injected abroad and their complications are also often managed in the United States as travelers return from overseas.[4] Thus, awareness of the potential types of complications and options for management, in addition to the underlying facial anatomy, are imperative to delivering the best patient care.

The importance of hyaluronidase is being mentioned early in this article because of its value in treating a variety of the complications of facial fillers. Hyaluronidase has the ability to dissolve HA, which comprises most fillers injected in the United States.[1] Its activity was first described in 1929 by Duran-Reynals.[5] It is FDA-approved as a dispersion agent, usually for local anesthetics, which temporarily modifies the permeability of connective tissue through the hydrolysis of HA, a polysaccharide found in the intracellular ground substance of connective tissue.[6] It is not FDA-approved for dissolution of HA and therefore use

Disclosures: Allergan, Galderma, Merz Aesthetics, Skin Ceuticals, Suneva (J. Woodward). None (T. Khan, J. Martin).
[a] Duke University Medical Center, Durham, NC, USA; [b] Duke University Medical Center, Coral Gables, FL, USA
[*] Corresponding author. Duke University Medical Center, 2351 Erwin Road, Durham, NC 27705.
E-mail address: Julie.woodward@duke.edu

facialplastic.theclinics.com

in treating complications from facial fillers is considered off-label.

Hyaluronidase has been used in ophthalmology with retrobulbar blocks since 1978.[7] It is commercially available in the United States as Vitrase (ovine from Valeant) and Hylenex (human recombinant from Halozyme).[6] Hyaluronidase has even been suggested as a possibility to treat non-HA fillers with the idea that increased tissue compliance may allow a non-HA emboli to pass. Approximately 30 U of hyaluronidase are needed to dissolve 0.1 mL of HA. Restylane may resolve the fastest and Belotero the slowest relative to more cross-linking in the latter.[8] All HA fillers, however, should be degraded within 24 hours.[9]

POOR COSMETIC RESULTS

Overfilled lips and nasolabial folds do not convey an aesthetically pleasing, natural, or rejuvenated face (**Fig. 1**). To create visually favorable results, facial fillers are often injected off-label in nonapproved facial regions. Although most fillers are FDA-approved only for nasolabial folds, Restylane and Restylane Silk are approved for lip augmentation, Juvederm Voluma for midface restoration, Sculptra and Radiesse for facial lipoatrophy, and Bellafil for acne scar modification.[2,3] Radiesse is soon to be approved for hand rejuvenation.

Nodules can be noninflammatory or inflammatory. A noninflammatory nodule caused by too much filler in a certain location can be disintegrated with vigorous massage, dissolved with hyaluronidase, or even extruded with needle puncture by expressing the filler material out of the dermal tissue. Lumps and bumps from overfilling in a particular area often respond to simple massage. If they do not subside within 1 to 2 weeks, they can be dissolved with hyaluronidase.

Fillers also have the potential to migrate from the intended area of treatment.[10,11] Experienced injectors are attuned to observing filler track along tissue planes away from the site of a needle entry. Filler material can migrate to the inside of the lip (**Fig. 2**) or from a nasolabial fold down toward the vermilion border (Niamtu Cohen, personal communication, 2013).

A blue-tinted hue is often described with HA fillers and termed the Tyndall effect. The phenomenon describes multidirectional light scattering from particles in a colloid dispersion. Blue light is scattered more strongly and this color can become visible as the light passes through boluses of nonhomogenous filler within the skin. The term, despite its classic association with dermal fillers, may not actually be the proper term for this phenomenon because the molecules are too large for this to occur.[12] The true mechanism is yet to be elucidated. If this bluish hue is noticeable, the skin can often be punctured with a needle to express the nodule of filler without any complication (**Fig. 3**). Topical antibiotic should be applied immediately afterward.

Delayed edema surrounding areas of HA injection is a notable phenomenon because of its hydrophilic nature and osmolality. Juvederm tends to attract more edema than other products.[13] Griepentrog and colleagues[14] reported that about one in four patients with Restylane injected into tear troughs experienced some degree of perceptible edema.[15]

Chronic prolonged edema can also be related to a type 4 hypersensitivity reaction. If it is unresponsive to antihistamines, it may need to be dissolved with hyaluronidase (**Figs. 4–6**). Angioedema is an immediate allergic response that can last for several weeks. It may respond to antihistamines or prednisone.[16]

Bruising is a complication of any procedure that involves the use of a needle or cannula. There is debate as to whether or not one should stop anticoagulants for patients receiving fillers.[17] For

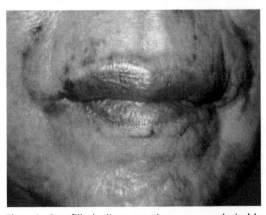

Fig. 1. Overfilled lips creating an undesirable aesthetic result.

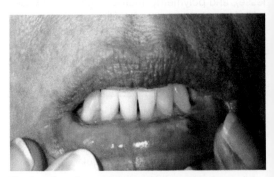

Fig. 2. Migration of filler material within lower lip.

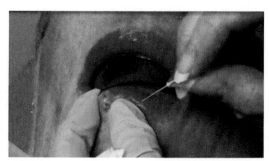

Fig. 3. Needle expression of retained filler material within lip.

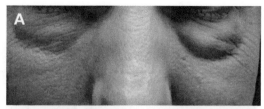

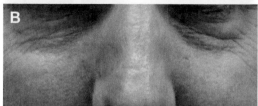

Fig. 5. Prolonged lower lid edema (*A*) improved with hyaluronidase treatment (*B*).

patients at low risk for cardiac disease or cerebrovascular disease, discontinuation of aspirin, nonsteroidal anti-inflammatory drugs, or herbal supplements, such as vitamin E, fish oil, ginseng, and ginkgo, is generally suggested. About 1.3% of the population may bruise because of a subclinical coagulopathy or von Willebrand disease. If a patient is at risk of thrombotic disease, the anticoagulants may be continued and the patient must be made aware of the increased risk of bruising.[16]

Some physicians believe that cannulas are safer and have less chance of causing bruising than needles. One double-blind randomized study demonstrated less side effects in the nasolabial fold with cannulas than with needles.[18]

Arnica montana is an herbal supplement that inhibits transcription factor nuclear factor-κB2 and has been promoted for its ability to minimize bruising. It can be applied topically, taken orally, or applied with a hydrogel deliver pad system along with Ledum (Cearna). The results have been controversial at best. Some dermatologists fear contact dermatitis from the topical form.[19] Oral *Arnica* demonstrated no improvement with blepharoplasty and hand surgery[20,21]; however, it did improve postoperative bruising associated with facelift procedures.[22] OcuMend has an

exclusive formula of *Arnica* that is 50 times more potent than all other *Arnica* products, and ledlum via its hydrogel delivery system. Studies are promising but yet to be reported in peer-reviewed literature.

Lastly, patients can suffer from vasovagal responses or seizures because of the stress of the injection procedure. Close supervision of the patient at all times and of physician extenders is recommended.

INFECTION: BIOFILMS

Proper topical preparation of the skin is inherently critical for prevention of infection. Topical alcohol 70% is inexpensive, readily available, and has quick onset. Topical chlorhexidine, available by swab or surgical scrub, is gaining popularity because it demonstrates a longer frame of action and tends to be nonirritating.[23]

Immediate bacterial infections are thought to be caused by introduction of bacteria from the

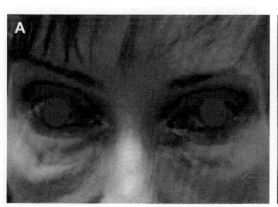

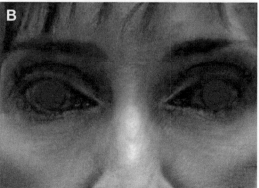

Fig. 4. Prolonged lower lid edema (*A*) improved with hyaluronidase treatment (*B*).

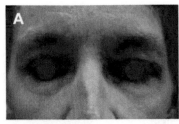
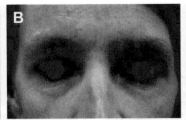
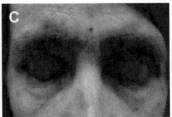

Fig. 6. Retained filler within upper lid (*A*) showing immediate improvement with hyaluronidase (*B*) and subsequently treated with additional filler for sulcus volume restoration (*C*).

surface of the skin though the injection portal sites. Such infections can often be treated with broad-spectrum oral antibiotics, such as clarithromycin (Biaxin), because of its activity against atypical mycobacteria.[24] Application of makeup should be delayed until 4 hours after injection. Reactivation of a herpetic infection is also possible and can be treated with oral valcyclovir, 2 to 3 g/day (**Fig. 7**).

Delayed infections caused by biofilms can be more difficult to treat. An inflamed nodule with a delayed presentation of 2 or more weeks can be caused by a biofilm. These can persist for months. A biofilm is an aggregate of self-encapsulated microorganisms in polymeric matrix, irreversibly adherent to a living or inert surface. Biofilms are difficult for oral antibiotics to penetrate, and they can be difficult to culture. They can contain bacteria, protozoa, or fungi in a low-grade infection that chronically seeds the local area and can even trigger a systemic infection.[25] Biofilms can be associated with foreign body granulomas (discussed in next section). Antibiotics should be started before any attempts to remove the granuloma with hyaluronidase (for HA); steroid, 40 mg/mL or fluorouracil (5-FU), 50 mg/mL injections; laser lysis; or surgical excision.[16] Infectious disease consultations may be

necessary for infections involving atypical mycobacteria or fungus.

GRANULOMAS

Foreign body granulomas present as inflamed red nodules that are culture negative (**Fig. 8**). Such a granuloma forms when activated macrophages engulf filler material and then secrete cytokines and inflammatory cytokines. These macrophages can coalesce to form multinucleated giant cells. Granulomatous reactions are rare and can present months to years after an injection. Intralesional steroids and 5-FU are the therapeutic mainstay to inhibit fibroblast activity. If the nodules are associated with an abscess, the infectious component is often sterile. Granulomas may occur more commonly with long-lasting or permanent fillers, such as silicone, polyacrylamide, PLLA, and PMMA.[16] Some of the granulomas caused by permanent fillers may take many years to present (**Fig. 9**).

Granuloma can be localized or present as a global systemic response (**Box 1**). All can be treated with use of hyaluronidase and oral or intravenous steroids. One patient experienced a global systemic reaction to HA that presented with bilateral ptosis (**Fig. 10**). Granulomas were noted in

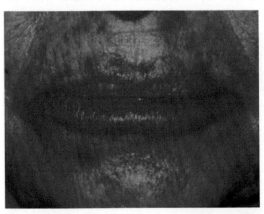

Fig. 7. Reactivation of oral herpes following filler treatment in the perioral region.

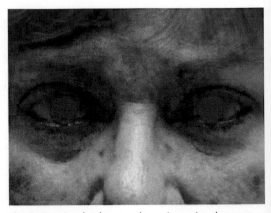

Fig. 8. Foreign body granuloma in periocular area.

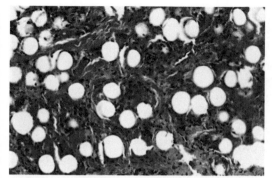

Fig. 9. Granulomatous response surrounding foreign filler material (hematoxylin-eosin, original magnification bar = 100 μm).

upper and lower eyelids, temples, cheeks, and lips. A test was placed on her forearm that reacted positive with granulomatous response (**Fig. 11**). The patient suffered knee and back pain possibly from cross reactivity with HA in her joints. After no improvement with antibiotics, she required hospital admission for intravenous methylprednisolone for 3 days followed by oral steroids for 1 month. All areas were dissolved with hyaluronidase on three occasions. One year after recovery, she was successfully treated with Belotero with no complications.

Box 1
Presentation and management of common filler complications

Nodules (early presentation)

- HA: extrusion, hyaluronidase
- Non-HA: intralesional steroids with lidocaine and/or 5-FU, microfocused ultrasound or fractional lasers, surgical excision

Inflammatory nodules

- Biofilm: antibiotics (biaxin, ciprofloxacin, or clarithromycin) for 4–6 weeks
- 5-FU 50 mg/mL, 0.1- to 0.5-mL injections
- Consider biopsy and infectious diseases consultation for atypical mycobacterium or fungus

Foreign body granulomas

- Localized: hyaluronidase if HA and intralesional steroids and/or 5-FU injections, then excision
- Global: hyaluronidase if HA, test spot on arm, biopsy, intralesional, or intravenous systemic steroids

---

VASCULAR OCCLUSION

One of the most devastating complications arising from facial filler injections is inadvertent intra-arterial embolization or from vascular compression, leading to localized skin necrosis or permanent vision loss (**Box 2**). Arterial embolization is more commonly direct anterograde with occlusion of an artery causing ischemia distal to the injection point. This direct form of occlusion usually occurs with injections to the glabellar region.[26] Clinically, patients manifest with significant pain and ischemic pallor, eventually leading to necrosis and atrophic changes. Hot compresses, massage, hyaluronidase, aspirin, and possibly oral steroids should be immediately considered.

A venous occlusion is also possible during cosmetic injections. Instead of immediate pain and blanching, this presents with venous mottling termed livido. Livido from venous occlusion should be distinguished from bruising. This patient was successfully treated with heat, massage, hyaluronidase, and prednisone (**Fig. 12**). Again, this can be treated with hyaluronidase, heat, massage, and oral steroids.

Retrograde flow of facial filler against arterial pressure to an arterial bifurcation followed by anterograde flow through the branch artery causes embolia cutis medicamentosa (also known as Freudenthal-Nicolau syndrome.) In this phenomenon, the anterograde flow is often through the ophthalmic artery and the central retinal artery to subsequently cause a vascular occlusion in the retina and thus blindness. The literature has described devastating permanent visual loss from injections of steroids in the head and neck region for various benign lesions (ie, chalazion, capillary hemangioma).[27,28] The substance must be injected against the systemic arterial pressure to fill the entire vessel retrograde past the bifurcation before it flows anterograde into the central retinal artery or its distal tributaries. Egbert and colleagues[29] approximated as little as 0.01 mL as the minimum required volume to cause vascular occlusion in the setting of intralesional corticosteroid injections to eyelid lesions. The volume of the supratrochlear artery has been assessed from cadaver head studies in which the supratrochlear artery was dissected anteriorly from the level of the glabella to the orbital apex. This calculated volume was measured as 0.085 mL (**Fig. 13**).[30]

Numerous case reports describe this retrograde occlusive event clinically arising from filler injections in the nasal dorsum, nasolabial folds,

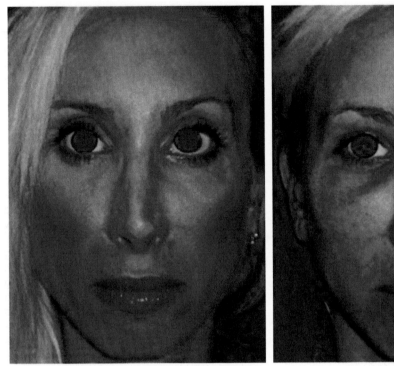
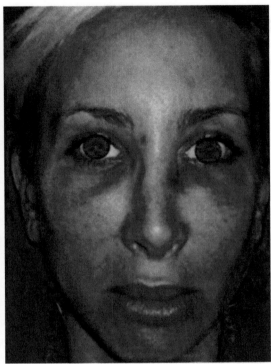

Fig. 10. Patient who experienced systemic adverse response to hyaluronic acid filler and with bilateral ptosis.

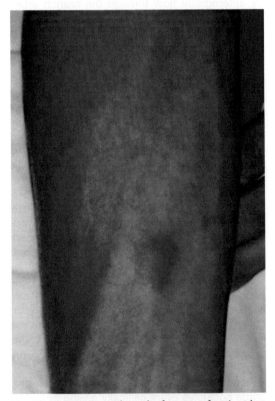

Fig. 11. Test response along the forearm of patient (see Fig. 10) demonstrating positive granulomatous reaction.

and lips.[31–34] The injected material typically enters the supratrochlear, supraorbital, or dorsal nasal artery (**Fig. 14**). It can then travel far posteriorly into the ophthalmic artery (a direct branch of the internal carotid artery), causing more dramatic, diffuse visual loss. A more anterograde occlusion of the central retinal artery (branch of the ophthalmic artery) would result in infarction of the anterior retinal layers, causing compromise of central visual acuity. Lastly, the anterograde flow may lodge the embolus into the posterior ciliary arteries or pial vasculature, which directly supply the optic nerve head and choroid.

When such a vascular event occurs, patients can immediately experience significant pain, skin blanching, loss of vision, and decreased extraocular motility. Rapid recognition of these symptoms can allow the injector to promptly manage the evolving vaso-occlusion with the following measures: applying pressure to the injection site in an effort to dislodge the embolus, injecting hyaluronidase (if an HA filler was used) to dissolve the filler particles, and applying nitroglycerin paste and topical oxygen therapy to allow for vasodilatation and spontaneous release of the occlusive bolus. Some sources, however, indicate that nitroglycerin paste may worsen the impending ischemia by propagating the filler

Box 2
Vascular occlusive events: presentation, treatment, and prevention

Venous

- Presentation: livido, lack of significant pain
- Treatment: heat, massage, oral prednisone, hyaluronidase if HA
- Prevention: awareness of anatomy danger zones, consider injection with cannulas, aspiration before injection, slow retrograde injections, avoid bolus injections greater than 0.1 mL

Arterial

Anterograde

- Presentation: pain, blanching distal to site of injection
- Treatment: heat, massage, aspirin, hyaluronidase, oxygen infusion cream, hyperbaric oxygen
- Prevention: awareness of anatomy danger zones, consider injection with cannulas, aspiration before injection, slow retrograde injections, avoid bolus injections greater than 0.1 mL

Retrograde followed by anterograde

- Presentation: dizziness, blindness, cerebrovascular accident, pain
- Treatment: heat, massage, acetylsalicylic acid (aspirin), hyaluronidase, hyperbaric oxygen
- Prevention: awareness of anatomy danger zones, consider injection with cannulas, aspiration before injection, slow retrograde injections, avoid bolus injections greater than 0.1 mL

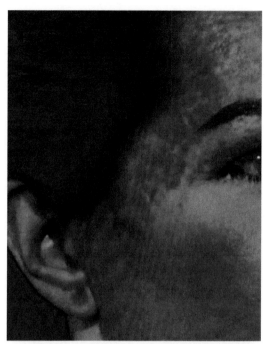

Fig. 12. Livido reticularis resulting from venous obstruction.

essential to increase the likelihood of a favorable result. HA fillers can be used in several different regions of the face and boast reversibility with the use of hyaluronidase. Semipermanent fillers, such as PMMA and PLLA, may offer greater facial scaffolding for patients who require more significant volume restoration; however,

substance into other portions of the arterial tree.[35]

Studies have consistently demonstrated that visual loss resulting from diffuse occlusions of the ophthalmic artery is more likely to occur with autologous fat injections because a greater volume is often necessary to overcorrect facial hollow deformities and therefore requires a larger needle to inject.[36] Additionally, fat is more likely to cause an embolus, whereas HA filler attracts water, which may prevent further particle migration.

PREVENTION

As with any procedure, proper patient selection and choice of method and/or product is

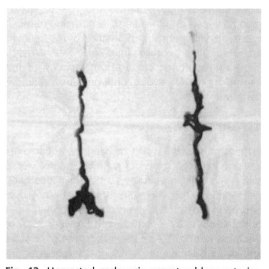

Fig. 13. Harvested cadaveric supratrochlear arteries. Average volume from glabella to orbital apex calculated as 0.085 mL.

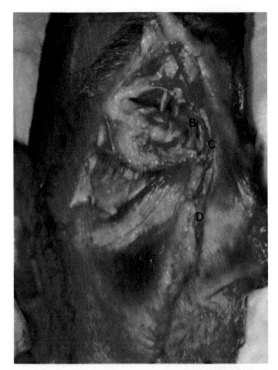

Fig. 14. Anatomic danger zones. (*A*) Supraorbital artery and nerve. (*B*) Supratrochlear artery. (*C*) Dorsal nasal artery. (*D*) Angular artery.

they cannot be easily corrected in the event of product migration or localized granulomatous reaction.

The method of injection also contributes to the overall result. Slower injection of smaller volumes generally less than 0.1 mL in any given location allows for more controlled filling. Injection by blunt cannula may minimize the risk of perforating a vessel and facilitates remodeling of facial ligaments with gentle manipulation of the cannula tip. Aspiration before injection can provide important anatomic clues about location of the needle tip and avoid unnecessary vascular penetration.

ILLEGAL FILLERS

In many parts of the world, the illegal injection market continues to grow as patients search for a quick, low-cost procedure to obtain a cosmetic rejuvenation. The injections are usually not performed in a medical setting but are done in spas or hotel rooms by a nonlicensed provider. One of the most popular illegal fillers is a type of silicone known as biopolymer. Although the patients are told that this is a medical-grade product, it is usually an industrial-grade, nonsterile type of silicone, often mixed with a variety of nonsterile products,

such as glycerin and polyacrylamide gel. Some injections have no silicone, but just the polyacrylamide gel, glycerin, and even reports of cement and fix-a-flat. Although the initial result may be cosmetically pleasing, with time the filler can migrate and cause a multitude of cosmetic and medical complications. These include granulomas, chronic local and systemic inflammation, inflammatory pulmonary disease, and blindness.[37–43] In addition, acute consequences, such as silicone embolus and death, have been reported.[44–50]

The use of liquid silicone for soft tissue augmentation has been practiced for many years. It has certain properties that theoretically make it a good filler: durability, resistance to heat, low immunogenicity, and noncarcinogenic. It also has a good cost to benefit ratio compared with other fillers. But silicone has also been associated with a high incidence of complications, many of which are caused by the volume injected. In the black market, a large volume of non-medical-grade silicone is often used by the unlicensed providers with volumes of up to 1 L being injected.[43]

Silicone granulomas are the most commonly reported side effect. The silicone may serve as a nidus for infection in the form of bacterial biofilms,[42] resulting in a recurrent cellulitis-like reaction with pain, induration, and nodules. Because this is a non-medical-grade substance, there may be foreign body reaction to adulterated product. The other products that are added to the silicone greatly increase the risk of foreign body reaction.

More serious adverse events, such as sepsis and silicone emboli resulting in death, have been reported. Factors associated with risk of silicone pulmonary embolism include the high pressure and large volume of the injections, and massage or trauma at the injection site postprocedure. The embolus can occur during or up to 24 hours after the injection.

Although some reactions occur within the first 72 hours, many of the serious adverse events can occur months to years postinjection, such as granulomatous nodules, ulceration, and cellulitis. Some patients develop open nonhealing sores, which can then lead to sepsis and death (**Fig. 15**).[40,41] Chen and colleagues[37] reported a granulomatous reaction that developed 40 years after facial silicone injection. Schmid and colleagues[46] reported 33 cases of "silicone syndrome" that occurred 24 to 72 hours postinjection. Most patients developed symptoms and signs consistent with pulmonary embolism: dyspnea, fever, cough, hemoptysis, chest pain,

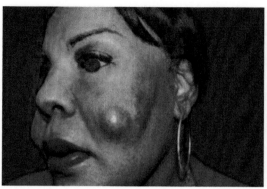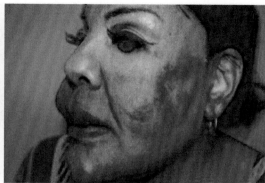

Fig. 15. Granulomatous nodule related to silicone filler injection.

hypoxia, and alveolar hemorrhage. There were eight deaths, two from pulmonary embolism and six from cerebral embolism.

The illegal silicone and other fillers are of low viscosity, which allows them to migrate. This can result in the development of distant deformities. In the face the filler can move from the cheek down into the jowls and neck with marked disfigurement of the face. After more than a microdroplet of silicone has been injected it infiltrates multiple tissue planes. This makes the eventual treatment extremely difficult. Small nodules can be surgically excised, but larger ones, similar to the ones described here, are very difficult to remove. When attempting to excise, the nodules can present as large sheets of hard subcutaneous tissue, or rocklike nodules, which are impossible to cut through (**Fig. 16**). When removing these nodules, one must excise all the tissue that has been infiltrated, leaving a large defect devoid of any normal tissue. Pathology examination performed on this tissue reveals the reactive changes that are occurring to the foreign material, but is unable to give a definitive diagnosis as to what was injected.

Other treatments that have been used to treat the inflammatory nodules from illegal fillers include steroid and 5-FU injections,[4] minocycline 100 twice daily,[51,52] and topical 5% imiquimod cream for lip nodules.[53]

In 2012 Kornstein first reported using microfocused ultrasound for silicone nodules in the lips. Multiple sessions are necessary.[54] The microfocused ultrasound can penetrate to 4.5 mm below the skin. This deep heating may break up and destroy or melt some of the fibrotic tissue in the nodules, which allows the body to better eliminate the granulomatous tissue (**Fig. 17**).

Despite the large amount of written and television press about the dangers of illegal silicone, many individuals still seek an inexpensive rejuvenation. It is hoped that educating the public of the very serious health risks involved in allowing nonlicensed injectors to use black market fillers results in fewer people seeking these horribly disfiguring treatments.

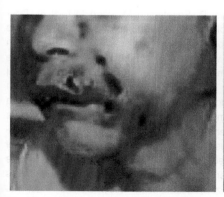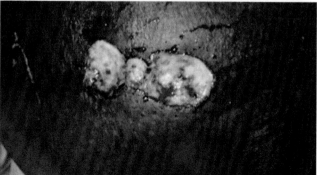

Fig. 16. Surgical excision of firm subcutaneous nodule resulting from silicone filler injection.

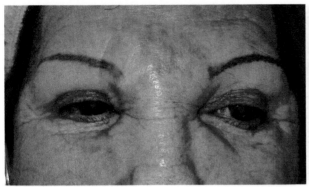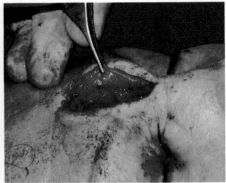

Fig. 17. Fibrotic forehead nodule that was surgically excised.

REFERENCES

1. American Society of Plastic Surgeons. 2013 Plastic Surgery Statistics Report. Available at: http://www.plasticsurgery.org/Documents/news-resources/statistics/2013-statistics/cosmetic-procedure-trends-2014.pdf. Accessed April 6, 2015.
2. United States Food and Drug Administration. Dermal Fillers Approved by the Center for Devices and Radiological Health. Available at: http://www.fda.gov/MedicalDevices/ProductsandMedicalProcedures/CosmeticDevices/WrinkleFillers/ucm227749.htm. Accessed April 6, 2015.
3. Physicians Coalition for Injectable Safety. Available at: www.injectablesafety.org. Accessed April 6, 2015.
4. Munro D, Ehrlic M, Woodward J. Successful management of delayed-onset complications from a dermal filler of unknown provenance. Am J Cosmet Surg 2013;30(4):235–8.
5. Duran-Reynals F. The effects of extracts of certain organs from normal and immunized animals on the infecting power of vaccine virus. J Exp Med 1929; 50:327–40.
6. Rzany B, Becker-Wegerich P, Bachmann F, et al. Hyaluronidase in the correction of hyaluronic acid-based fillers: a review and a recommendation for use. J Cosmet Dermatol 2009;8:317–23.
7. Mindel JS. Value of hyaluronidase in ocular surgical akinesia. Am J Ophthalmol 1978;85:643–6.
8. Rao V, Chi S, Woodward J. Reversing facial fillers: interactions between hyaluronidase and commercially available hyaluronic-acid based fillers. J Drugs Dermatol 2014;13(9):1053–6.
9. Flynn TC, Thompson DH, Hyun SH, et al. Ultrastructural analysis of 3 hyaluronic acid soft-tissue fillers using scanning electron microscopy. Dermatol Surg 2015;41(Suppl 1):S143–52.
10. Jordan DR, Stoica B. Filler migration: a number of mechanisms to consider. Ophthal Plast Reconstr Surg 2015;31(4):257–62.
11. De Boulle K. Management of complications after implantation of fillers. J Cosmet Dermatol 2004; 3(1):2–15.
12. Rootman DB, Lin JL, Goldberg R. Does the Tyndall effect describe the blue hue periodically observed in subdermal hyaluronic acid gel placement? Ophthal Plast Reconstr Surg 2014;30(6): 524–7.
13. Tzikas TL. Chapter 18: soft tissue fillers for facial augmentation. In: Fedok FG, Carniol PJ, editors. Minimally invasive and office-based procedures in facial plastic surgery. Thieme; 2013.
14. Griepentrog GJ, Lucarelli MJ, Burkat CN, et al. Periorbital edema following hyaluronic acid gel injection: a retrospective review. Am J Cosmet Surg 2011; 28(4):251–4.
15. Morris CL, Stinnett SS, Woodward JA. Patient-preferred sites of Restylane injection in periocular and facial soft-tissue augmentation. Ophthal Plast Reconstr Surg 2008;24(2):117–21.
16. Funt D, Pavicic T. Dermal fillers in aesthetics: an overview of adverse events and treatment approaches. Clin Cosmet Investig Dermatol 2013;6: 295–316.
17. Zeichner JA, Cohen JL. Dermal fillers in patients on anticoagulants. J Drugs Dermatol 2010;9(9): 1059–60.
18. Hexsel D, Soirefmann M, Porto MD, et al. Double-blind, randomized, controlled clinical trial to compare safety and efficacy of a metallic cannula with that of a standard needle for soft tissue augmentation of the nasolabial folds. Dermatol Surg 2012;38(2):207–14.
19. Waldorf H. Maximizing filler results. Presentation at: Cosmetic Surgery Forum. Las Vegas (NV), December 5, 2014.
20. Kotlus BS, Heringer DM, Dryden RM. Evaluation of homeopathic *Arnica montana* for ecchymosis after upper blepharoplasty: a placebo-controlled, randomized, double-blind study. Ophthal Plast Reconstr Surg 2010;26(6):395–7.

21. Stevinson C, Devaraj VS, Fountain-Barber A, et al. Homeopathic *Arnica* for prevention of pain and bruising: randomized placebo-controlled trial in hand surgery. J R Soc Med 2003;96(2):60–5.

22. Seeley BM, Denton AB, Ahn MS, et al. Effect of homeopathic *Arnica montana* on bruising in face-lifts: results of a randomized, double-blind, placebo-controlled clinical trial. Arch Facial Plast Surg 2006;8(1):54–9.

23. Bailey SH, Cohen JL, Kenkel JM. Etiology, prevention, and treatment of dermal filler complications. Aesthet Surg J 2011;31(1):110–21.

24. Narins RS, Jewell M, Rubin M, et al. Clinical conference: management of rare events following dermal fillers–focal necrosis and angry red bumps. Dermatol Surg 2006;32(3):426–34.

25. Sadashivaiah AB, Mysore V. Biofilms: their role in dermal fillers. J Cutan Aesthet Surg 2010; 3(1):20–2.

26. Roberts SA, Arthurs BP. Severe visual loss and orbital infarction following periorbital aesthetic poly-(L)-lactic aci (PLLA) injection. Ophthal Plast Reconstr Surg 2012;28(3):68–70.

27. Edwards AO. Central retinal artery occlusion following forehead injection with a corticosteroid suspension. Pediatr Dermatol 2008;25(4):460–1.

28. McEwan G, Hofmeister E, Kubis K, et al. Monocular embolic retinal arteriolar occlusions after ipsilateral intraoral triamcinolone injection. J Neuroophthalmol 2010;30(1):98–9.

29. Egbert JE, Paul S, Engel WK, et al. High injection pressure during intralesional injection of corticosteroids into capillary hemangiomas. Arch Ophthalmol 2001;119:677–83.

30. Khan TT, Colon-Acevedo B, Woodward JA. An anatomical analysis of the supratrochlear artery and considerations in facial filler injections. Study in progress.

31. Lazzeri D, Agostini T, Figus M, et al. Blindness following cosmetic injections of the face. Plast Reconstr Surg 2012;129(4):995–1012.

32. Kwon SG, Hong JW, Roh TS, et al. Ischemic oculomotor nerve palsy and skin necrosis caused by vascular embolization after hyaluronic acid filler injection: a case report. Ann Plast Surg 2013;71(4): 333–4.

33. Park SH, Sun HJ, Choi KS. Sudden unilateral visual loss after autologous fat injection into the nasolabial fold. Clin Ophthalmol 2008;2(3): 679–83.

34. Kim SN, Byun DS, Park JH, et al. Panophthalmoplegia and vision loss after cosmetic nasal dorsum injection. J Clin Neurosci 2014;21(4): 678–80.

35. Hwang CJ, Morgan PV, Pimentel A, et al. Rethinking the role of nitroglycerin ointment in ischemic vascular filler complications: an animal model with ICG imaging. Ophthal Plast Reconstr Surg 2015. [Epub ahead of print].

36. Park KH, Kim YK, Woo SJ, et al. Iatrogenic occlusion of the ophthalmic artery after cosmetic facial filler injections: a national survey by the Korean Retina Society. JAMA Ophthalmol 2014;132(6): 714–23.

37. Chen YC, Chen ML, Chiu YM. A case of mimicking angioedema: chin silicone granulomatous reaction spreading all over the face after receiving liquid silicon e injection forty years previously. Chin Med J 2011;124(11):1747–50.

38. Altmeyer MD, Anderson LL, Wang AR. Silicone migration and granuloma formation. J Cosmet Dermatol 2009;8(2):92–7.

39. Tangsirichaipong A. Blindness after facial contour augmentation with injectable silicone. J Med Assoc Thai 2009;92(Suppl 3):S85–7.

40. Essenmacher AC, Astani SA. Respiratory disease following illicit injection of silicone. A case report. Case Rep Med 2013;2013:743–842.

41. Seward AC, Meara DJ. Industrial-grade silicone injections causing intermittent bilateral malar swelling. J Oral Maxillofac Surg 2013;71(7):1245–8.

42. Duffy DM. The silicone conundrum: a battle of anecdotes. Dermatol Surg 2002;28:590–4.

43. Chastre J, Brun P, Soler P, et al. Acute and latent pneumonitis after subcutaneous injections of silicone in transsexual men. Am Rev Respir Dis 1987; 135:236–40.

44. Restrepo CS, Artunduaga M, Carrillo JA, et al. Silicone pulmonary embolism: report of 10 cases and review of the literature. J Comput Assist Tomogr 2009;33(2):233–7.

45. Price EA, Schueler H, Perper JA. Massive systemic silicone embolism: a case report and review of the literature. Am J Forensic Med Pathol 2006; 27:97–102.

46. Schmid A, Tzur A, Leshko L, et al. Silicone embolism syndrome: a case report, review of the literature and comparison with fat embolism syndrome. Chest 2005;127:2276–81.

47. Orentrich DS. Liquid injectable silicone techniques for soft tissue augmentation. Clin Plast Surg 2000; 27:595–612.

48. Hevia O. Six year experience using 1,000-centistoke silicone oil in 916 patients for soft-tissue augmentation in a private practice setting. Dermatol Surg 2009;35(Suppl 2):1646–52.

49. Fulton JE, Porumb S, Caruso JC, et al. Lip augmentation with liquid silicone. Dermatol Surg 2005;31(11 Pt2):1577–85.

50. Moscona RA, Fodor L. A retrospective study on liquid injectable silicone for lip augmentation: long-term results and patient satisfaction. J Plast Reconstr Aesthet Surg 2010;63(10): 1694–8.

51. Senet P, Bachelez H, Ollivaud L, et al. Minocycline for treatment of cutaneous silicone granulomas. Br J Dermatol 1999;140:985.

52. Arin MJ, Bäte J, Krieg T, et al. Silicone granuloma of the face treated with minocycline. J Am Acad Dermatol 2005;52(2 Suppl 1):53–6.

53. Baumann LS, Halem ML. Lip silicone granulomatous foreign body reaction treated with aldara (imiquimod 5%). Dermatol Surg 2003; 29(4):429–32.

54. Kornstein AN. Ulthera for silicone lip correction. Plast Reconstr Surg 2012;129(6):1014e–5e.

Collagen Stimulators
Poly-L-Lactic Acid and Calcium Hydroxyl Apatite

Andrew Breithaupt, MD, Rebecca Fitzgerald, MD*

KEYWORDS

- Collagen stimulators • Calcium hydroxyl apatite • Poly-L-lactic acid • Facial rejuvenation • Fillers

KEY POINTS

- Aging is a three-dimensional process, with changes in multiple tissues contributing to the overall effect.
- The role of volume loss in the clinical changes observed in the aging face is becoming widely appreciated. Mastery of volume replacement has become essential to the successful practice of aesthetic medicine.
- Lifting techniques alone, without addressing volume loss, can no longer adequately address the aging process in the face. This approach may actually exacerbate, rather than ameliorate, the aging process.
- Calcium hydroxyl apatite and poly-L-lactic acid, the so-called collagen stimulators, offer a unique and effective way to address this issue with natural-appearing results with long duration.

 Videos of dorsal hand treatment with calcium hydroxyl appetite; and panfacial treatment with poly-L-lactic acid accompany this article at http://www.facialplastic.theclinics.com/

INTRODUCTION

Over the last decade, many studies of the structural changes observed in the aging face (in bone, fat pads, facial ligaments, muscle, skin) have increased our understanding that facial rejuvenation is far more complex and nuanced than simply filling lines and folds or cutting and lifting soft tissue and skin.[1-3] This, in addition to the many new products introduced to the marketplace over the same time period has fueled our evolution of panfacial rejuvenation and restoration using fillers.[4]

According to the American Society of Plastic Surgeons (ASPS), more than 1.7 million injections

of soft tissue filler were performed in the United States in 2014 alone. This represents more than a 250% increase from just 14 years ago. Most of these injections used hyaluronic acid (HA)-based products, however close to a quarter of a million of these injections were carried out over the year using calcium hydroxylapatite (CaHA) (Radiesse, Merz Pharma, Frankfurt, Germany) and poly-L-lactic acid (PLLA) (Sculptra, Sinclair Pharmaceuticals, Galderma Laboratories, Fort Worth, TX, USA).[5]

The purpose of this article is to discuss current techniques used with CaHA and PLLA to safely and effectively address the changes observed in the aging face. The original US Food and Drug Administration (FDA) studies for aesthetic approval

Disclosures: None (A. Breithaupt); Speaker, Trainer, Consultant, and Advisory Board Member for Allergan, Merz, Galderma, and Valeant (R. Fitzgerald).
Department of Medicine, David Geffen School of Medicine, University of California, Los Angeles, Los Angeles, CA, USA
* Corresponding author. Private Practice, 321 North Larchmont Boulevard, Suite 906, Los Angeles, CA 90004.
E-mail address: fitzmd@earthlink.net

of most of the currently commercially available fillers, including these 2, looked at correction of the nasolabial fold by direct injection using a recognized and standardized grading chart and then subsequently gave approval for "subdermal implantation for the correction of moderate to severe facial wrinkles and folds, such as nasolabial folds." These 2 products also received FDA approval for restoration and/or correction of the signs of facial fat loss (lipoatrophy) in people with human immunodeficiency virus. More recently, in 2015, Radiesse was approved by the FDA for dorsal hand augmentation. On-label refers to use strictly as described in the studies carried out to garner FDA approval (and these are the only uses for which the product manufacturers may commercially promote their product). With time and experience, doctors may discover other advantageous uses of these products, and this is referred to as off-label use. Many of the techniques described in this article are off-label.

Much has already been written about the science behind these products. A brief review follows here.

The principal component of Radiesse is CaHA, a biomaterial with more than 20 years of safe and effective use for devices in orthopedics, neurosurgery, dentistry, otolaryngology, and ophthalmology, demonstrating its biocompatibility and low incidence of allergenicity.[6] Calcium hydroxylapatite is a synthetic analogue of the inorganic constituent of bone and teeth. The CaHA microspheres (25–45 μm) represent 30% of the final product and are suspended in a 70% gel carrier containing sterile water, carboxymethylcellulose, and glycerin. An immediate fill and lift is seen from the gel carrier, which dissipates over the next several weeks, while the CaHA remains at the site of injection. When this site is examined 3 months later, the CaHA microspheres are encapsulated by a network of fibrin, fibroblasts, and macrophages, with the CaHA acting as a scaffolding for fibroplasia and new collagen formation. At 9 months, the microspheres begin to absorb and can be found within macrophages.[7] The clinical result can last for 12 to 18 months. The glycerin helps the product flow from the syringe, but may cause pronounced transient swelling and edema. The patient should be made aware that this swelling is only temporary (24–72 hours).

One method used to help select the optimum product for a specific area (ie, soft product for lips, stiff product for chin) is to look at a given product's rheology. Rheology is the study of the flow characteristics of different products (eg, cement vs water); one rheological component that can be measured is referred to as G′. G′ is a measure

of elasticity, meaning a material's stiffness or ability to resist deformation under pressure. Radiesse has a high G′ value, which is suitable for lifting soft tissue and contouring, making it an ideal agent, for example, for deep supra-periosteal injections along the malar eminence and zygomatic arch, the mandible, and the chin.[8] This can be done to replenish volume in areas of bony remodeling in an aged face, or to create bony prominence in patients with congenital skeletal hypoplasia.

The product can also be diluted and used to augment the dorsal hand.[9]

PLLA is a synthetic, biocompatible, and biodegradable polymer of lactic acid that has been used safely in various medical applications for more than 3 decades.[10] The product is supplied as a lyophilized powder in a sterile glass vial and includes nonpyrogenic mannitol, sodium carboxymethylcellulose, and PLLA microparticles (40–60 μm). The product must be reconstituted with sterile water before injection and this is discussed in more detail later. A transient fill as a result of the mechanical distention of the tissues is seen immediately after injection, but this resorbs over the next several days. The true mechanism of action of PLLA begins with a subclinical inflammatory tissue response after implantation, followed by encapsulation of the particles and subsequent fibroplasia. This fibroplasia volumizes the tissues and produces the desired cosmetic result. This mechanism of action enables the product to gradually and progressively restore "a little volume all over" yielding a subtle and natural-looking result. It is important for both the practitioner and the patient to note that the final result is not accomplished by the product, but by the host's reaction to the product, and that this process takes 3 to 4 weeks.[10]

The bioengineering definition of biocompatibility is "the ability to elicit an appropriate host reaction in a desired application."[11] In the application of tissue augmentation, this requires a predictable amount of inflammation. A predictable amount of inflammation (and therefore a predictable result) is easily achievable by avoiding overcorrection. A predictable amount of inflammation requires 3 things: (1) a predictable product (with a homogeneous particle size), (2) a predictable methodology (achieved over the last decade of use), and (3) a predictable patient (the absence of active autoimmune disease).[12] As experience has been gained with this product and technical issues have evolved, we have seen that most of the adverse events seen with early use (papules and nodules, especially around the eyes or lips), stemmed from suboptimal technique. Therefore, a few simple yet critical components of methodology unique to this product (product reconstitution, placement, and treatment intervals) are worth mentioning here. The common denominator is an even distribution of product and avoidance of overcorrection.[13,14] Current reconstitution recommendations are a dilution of more than 5 mL (most experienced practitioners recommend a 9 mL dilution) and a hydration time of at least 2 hours (most experienced practitioners recommend more than 24 hours). The product should not be splashed up onto the side walls of the vial (by adding the water with too much force or shaking after addition of water) as this product will not be properly hydrated. Injection of poorly hydrated product leads to in vivo hydration of a clump of product and this leads to nodules.

Placement precautions include avoidance of superficial placement (may lead to visible fibroplasia), as well as placement in or through active muscles particularly around the eye or lip (which leads to nodules representing product trapped in muscle fibers).[12–14]

The final fill is achieved not by the product but by the host reaction to the product and, as this takes time, this is done incrementally. This means the end point of any one treatment session is not full visual correction, but simply to blanket the area to be treated and is determined solely and completely by the amount of surface area to be treated at that session using approximately 0.1 to 0.3 mL/cm^2 when using a subcutaneous fanning or crosshatch technique or 0.3 to 0.5 mL/cm^2 to place supraperiosteal depots followed by vigorous massage. The final volumetric correction is determined by the number of treatment sessions. Treatment intervals should be a minimum of 4 weeks, longer in younger or fuller faces, or those nearing their treatment goal in order to prevent a fat face. This means for example, that a large face with only mild volume loss may require 3 vials/session but only 1 session, whereas a small face with severe lipoatrophy may require only 2 vials/session but 3 or more sessions. Although patients in their 50s or 60s often need 3 sessions, a younger or fuller face may require only 1 or 2 vials/session and 1 or 2 sessions.[12–14] The longevity of the product makes this trouble worthwhile. In the study used to garner FDA aesthetic approval, almost 80% of the patients treated still saw full correction at 25 months (the cutoff time of the study).[15]

PREOPERATIVE PLANNING AND PREPARATION

As with any cosmetic procedure, the physician should set realistic expectations and review any possible complications (discussed later). Treatment of any patient who does not demonstrate sufficient understanding should be avoided. Patients treated with Radiesse should be forewarned that they may experience edema and swelling for 1 to 2 days. Patients treated with PLLA should be educated on the gradual onset of effects, the possible need for multiple sessions, and the long-lasting nature of the results.

The value of standardized photography cannot be overstated and should be used both to guide the treatment approach and to follow the results and plan future treatments.

During the evaluation of the patient, they should be viewed sitting upright from multiple angles. Normal facial animation can help to reveal areas of volume loss or rhytides that may not be found at rest. Having the patient lean over with their face toward the floor can also help accentuate volume loss, especially in the midface.

Most patients have lost a little integrity in multiple structural layers (skin, fat, or bone), but some have focal deficits in one tissue that outweighs the others. For example, after a facelift, the patient may have lost some volume in their peripheral face from atrophy of the temporal and lateral cheek fat, whereas after endurance exercise or in a young mom who just finished a year of breastfeeding, there may be loss of deep fat in the midface. A young patient with skeletal hypoplasia may just want augmentation of their cheekbones or chin, or to address their undereye hollows. An older patient often needs augmentation that mimics both bony and soft tissue. Evaluation of the tissue-specific loss (or absence) seen in the face in front of you at that point in time may yield better results than treating nasolabial folds or marionette lines in all comers. A schematic depiction of the superficial and deep fat pads, as well as one depicting areas of bony remodeling, are seen in **Figs. 1** and **2**. This recently described anatomy can be helpful in locating site-specific targets for treatment in different faces.[1,2]

Topical anesthesia can be applied before treatment. We use a betacaine/lidocaine/tetracaine mixture.

Antiseptic technique is imperative. We use a chlorhexidine scrub with sterile water followed by isopropyl alcohol immediately before injection. Surgical gloves should be changed if suspected of any contamination during the procedure (ie, touching the oral mucosa).

PATIENT POSITIONING

Treatment with PLLA is usually done with the patient sitting up. Radiesse in the cheeks or chin is administered with the patient in a semi-recumbent position. Radiesse is administered in

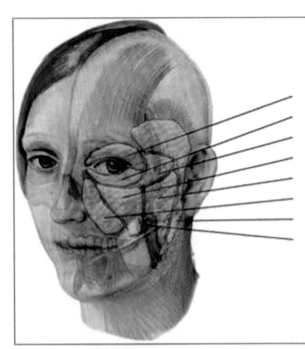

Superior orbital fat
Inferior orbital fat
Lateral orbital fat
Medial cheek fat
Middle cheek fat
Nasolabial fat
Lateral temporal-cheek fat
Buccal extension of the buccal fat

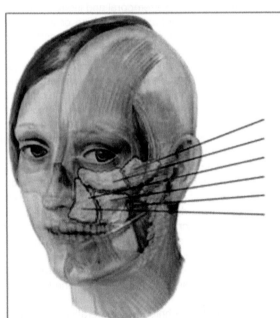

Sub–orbicularis oculi fat (lateral part)
Sub–orbicularis oculi fat (medial part)
Deep medial cheek fat (medial part)
Deep medial cheek fat (lateral part)
Buccal extension of the buccal fat
Ristow´s space

Fig. 1. The superficial and deep fat compartments. (*From* Gierloff M, Stöhring C, Buder T, et al. Aging changes of the midfacial fat compartments: a computed tomographic study. Plast Reconstr Surg 2012;129(1):263–73; with permission.)

the hands with the patient sitting up with their hands crossed over their lap.

These are really just issues of style and comfort, and can be done in a number of ways. The only thing that merits mention is that the supine position can change the draping of the soft tissues to be treated and this may be misleading.

PROCEDURAL APPROACH
Radiesse for Cheek and Chin Augmentation

We prefer to inject Radiesse with a 25-gauge cannula. First, a small dermal injection of 1% lidocaine is given with a 30-gauge needle. This needle is removed and if no brisk bleeding is noted, it is

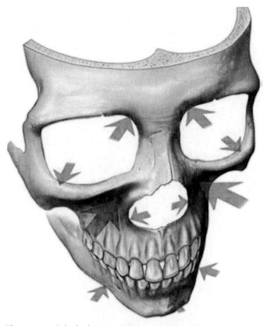

Fig. 2. Facial skeleton. Arrows indicate the areas of the facial skeleton susceptible to resorption with aging. The size of the arrow correlates with the amount of resorption. (*From* Mendelson B, Wong C. Changes in the facial skeleton with aging: implications and clinical applications in facial rejuvenation. Aesthetic Plast Surg 2012;36:753–60.)

replaced with a 22-gauge pilot needle inserted through the same opening just through the dermis. (If brisk bleeding is noted, firm pressure should be applied and another entry point created nearby.) This is then removed and replaced with a 25-gauge cannula attached to the syringe containing product. Note that the cannula is a two-dimensional instrument that can enter the dermis in the direction of the pilot needle only. Lateral traction on the skin at the insertion site can help ease insertion of the cannula into the skin.

The cannula is then inserted deeply, down to the periosteum, advanced forward along the bony surface to be treated, and then small aliquots are delivered slowly and evenly on withdrawal. This is continued in a fanning pattern until the desired area has been treated. The cannula should not be pushed forcefully through resistance (this can cause cannulas to enter blood vessels). Care is also taken not to redeposit product at the apex of a fan to avoid nodularity. In the cheek, over the zygomatic arch, this is done from 2 or 3 entry points that are either lateral or inferior to the apex of the bone. The amount of product required in this area varies from patient to patient, but is usually between 0.75 and 1.5 mL. The product can be molded into place after injection to ensure a smooth and even placement along the entire length of the zygoma. More product is placed at the superior aspect of the apex of the cheekbone to achieve a youthful anterior projection. For male patients, the product should be placed more inferiorly and laterally along the surface of the zygoma to avoid a feminizing look. If there is volume loss in the submalar/mid cheek where bony background is absent, the product should instead be placed in the deep subcutaneous plane. Superficial injections should be avoided to minimize the risk of nodule formation or lumpiness.

For treatment along the jawline, a cannula insertion point is created along the posterior aspect of the mandible as described earlier for the cheekbones. Again the plane of injection is deep (supraperiosteal). Product can be placed on the mandibular ramus alone or along the entire length of the mandible. It should be placed on both the anterior and inferior aspects to recreate the three-dimensional bony surface.

This same technique is used along the bone in the area of the prejowl sulcus, on both the anterior and inferior surface of the mandible. Product is also placed deeply (under the mentalis muscle) along the anterior and inferior surface of the chin. The body of the mentalis can be grasped and lifted away from the bone with the noninjecting hand while product is placed in the supraperiosteal plane. It is not uncommon to use 1.5 to 3 mL (1 syringe in the chin and prejowl sulcus, and one-half syringe along each mandibular border) in the lower face depending on the age and bone structure of the patient.

Before and after photographs of patients treated with this technique are shown in **Figs. 3–5**. The ASPS statistics referred to earlier have shown that "baby boomers", those aged 51 to 64 years, have traditionally accounted for the largest number of patients receiving these treatments. However, in the last 2 years, Gen-Xers, have taken over the lead. In 2014, people aged 35 to 50 years had the most procedures performed, over 4.2 million and 40.1% of the total, whereas people aged 51 to 64 years accounted for 31%.[5] For this reason, patients in this younger age group are also shown in these examples.

For rejuvenation of the hands, multiple techniques can be used. Because of the thin skin in this area, we prefer to use dilute product to avoid lumpiness and surface irregularities.

For this technique we dilute the product (which already contains lidocaine) with 1 mL of normal saline. A 25-gauge cannula is used in a manner similar to that described earlier. We use 1 of 2 possible entry points: the finger web spaces or the knuckles. The dorsal hand injection can also

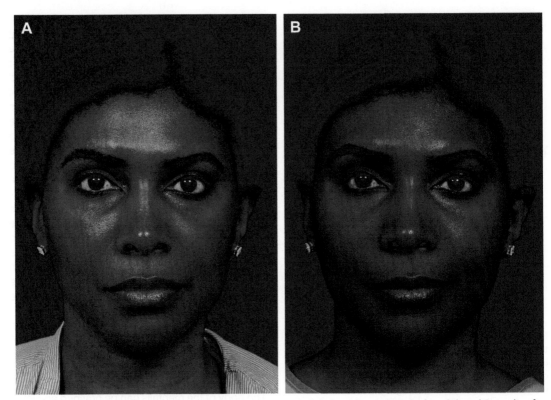

Fig. 3. A 38-year-old African American woman with congenital skeletal hypoplasia before (*A*) and 2 weeks after (*B*) 4.5-mL of calcium hydroxyl apatite filler (Radiesse). A total of 1.5 mL was used in the midface on each side, and 1.5 mL was used in the chin and the prejowl sulcus.

be carried out through an injection point in the proximal wrist. The cannula is placed into the plane just below the skin (above the vessels), between the tendons, and injected as a series of parallel fine thin threads in a fanning pattern on withdrawal of the cannula. Gentle massage is done after implantation. This technique is preferred over aggressive massage of 1 or 2 large depots of product because there is much less swelling noted. A narrated video demonstration of this technique is provided (Video 1; available online at http://www.facialplastic.theclinics.com/).

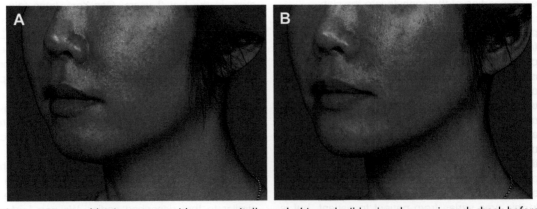

Fig. 4. A 42-year-old Asian woman with a congenitally weak chin and mild aging changes in each cheek before (*A*) and 4 weeks after (*B*) treatment with calcium hydroxyl apatite (Radiesse). A total of 1.5 mL was divided between each cheek, and 1.5 mL was used in the chin and prejowl sulcus.

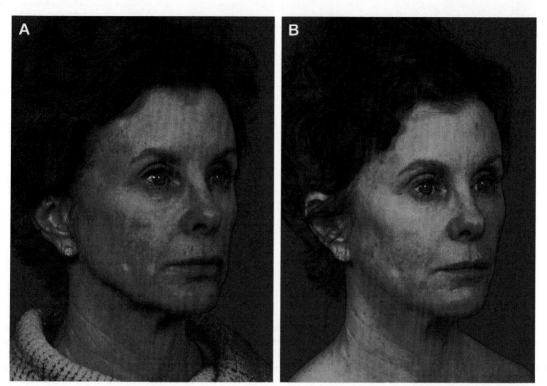

Fig. 5. A 55-year-old white woman with age-related volume loss before (*A*) and 4 weeks after (*B*) 6 mL of calcium hydroxyl apatite (Radiesse). A total of 3 mL was used on each side of the face; 1.5 mL was used along the zygomatic arch and 1.5 mL was used along the mandible, prejowl sulcus, and chin on each side of the face.

Panfacial Poly-ʟ-Lactic Acid

PLLA is hydrated with 8 mL of sterile water 24 to 72 hours before injection and 1 mL of 1% lidocaine is added immediately before injection. The suspension is shaken and mixed evenly and then drawn up into four 3-mL syringes each containing a bit more than 2 mL of product. The product may precipitate in the individual syringes before use and may then be mixed again immediately before injection by pulling 1 mL of air into the syringe and rotating it up and down (as shown in the video). The needle is then removed, any foam is pushed through the top of the syringe (the foam causes clogging), and the needle replaced and primed before injection. Constant clogging occurs when all of the foam is not expelled from the syringe and needle. The product is then injected with a 25-gauge 3.8-cm (1.5-inch) needle. Aspiration is carried out before every injection to avoid an inadvertent intravascular injection.

Depot injections of 0.5 to 1.0 mL are done on the bone in the temple, the canine fossa, and the chin. More than one depot may be used in a large empty temple. Fanning injections using 0.1 to 0.3 mL/cm² are placed deeply over the maxilla and zygomatic arch. Injections in the preauricular and lateral cheek area are done subcutaneously just under the skin (deeper injections in this area may enter the parotid gland or duct).

A video demonstration of this technique in a 41-year-old woman (Video 2 is available online at http://www.facialplastic.theclinics.com/) along with before and after photographs of the patient 1 month after treatment (**Fig. 6**). Additional examples of treatment using this technique can be seen in **Figs. 7–9**.

PLLA has been used in the dorsal hand and neck, however we avoid using it in these locations secondary to a relatively high rate of papule and nodule formation.[16] However, it is an excellent treatment for the décolleté area; this is done with a 16-mL dilution placed in a crosshatch fanning pattern over the area. A more detailed description is available elsewhere.[17]

POTENTIAL COMPLICATIONS AND MANAGEMENT

Potential complications can be divided into injection-related events, undesirable results from

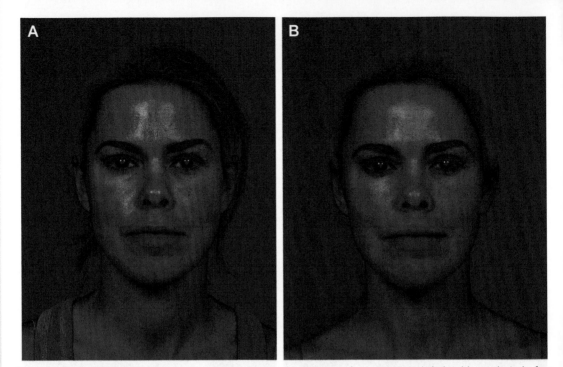

Fig. 6. A 41-year-old white woman with aging changes superimposed on congenital skeletal hypoplasia before (*A*) and 4 weeks after (*B*) 2 vials of poly-L-lactic acid used panfacially as demonstrated with narration in the video provided in this section. Neuromodulator was used in the glabella. Note the increased brow projection, bizygomatic width, and improvement in the perioral support giving an improved phi ratio to the lower third of the face as well as additional support to the soft tissue of the lips resulting in mild eversion of the upper and lower lip. Note also the ovalization of the facial shape. Some degree of improvement in the skin can be seen.

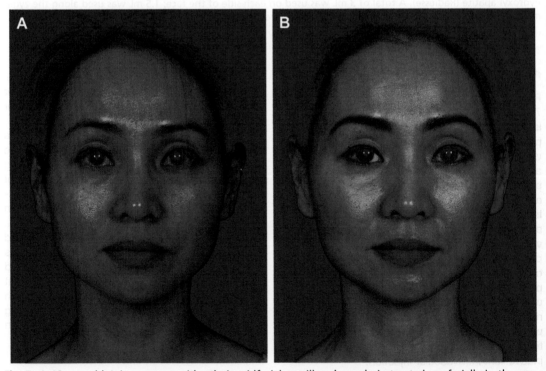

Fig. 7. A 46-year-old Asian woman with ethnic midfacial maxillary hypoplasia treated panfacially in the same manner as the patient in the video demonstration before (*A*) and 4 months after (*B*) 2 monthly sessions with 2 vials/session of poly-L-lactic acid. Note the subtle change in the position of the nose, and the mild eversion of the lips seen with treatment in the canine fossa. Again, some degree of skin improvement can be appreciated. This patient was also treated with neuromodulater in the glabellar area. On close observation of this photograph, this patient would likely benefit from calcium hydroxyl apatite treatment of the chin.

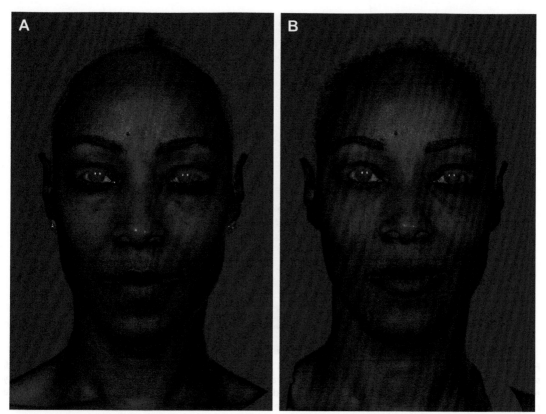

Fig. 8. A 48-year-old African American woman with ethnic midfacial maxillary hypoplasia treated panfacially in the same manner as the patient in the video demonstration before (*A*) and again 6 months after (*B*) 2 sessions with 2 vials/session of poly-L-lactic acid spaced 3 months apart. Again, note the subtle change in the position of the nose as well as the definition of the cheekbones. Some improvement is again noted in the skin. Neuromodulater was used in the glabellar area.

suboptimal technique, and true complications (which can be subdivided into inflammatory and vascular events).

The most common injection-related events are swelling, bruising, erythema, and pain, which resolve spontaneously over a short period of time. These can also be treated with acetomenophin, nonsteroidal antiinflammatory drugs, and cold compresses.

The most common consequence of suboptimal technique with these agents are papules and nodules. As these represent an overabundance of product (as opposed to a true granuloma, which represents an overabundance of host reaction to product), treatment with steroids or antimetabolites such as 5-fluorouracil will not resolve the problem. Intralesional steroids may, in fact, exacerbate the problem by causing atrophy around the site and making the lesions more noticeable. Excision is an option but trades a permanent scar for a transient problem. Camouflage with hyaluronic acid until the product resorbs is a viable option. The incidence of these events has decreased sharply as our understanding of the mechanism of action of these agents has improved and informed our techniques.[16]

The most common inflammatory complication with PLLA and Radiesse are clinical granulomas. Clinical granulomas represent an overabundance of host reaction to product, appear in all treated sites simultaneously, and have been reported with all commercially available fillers. Clinical granulomas are an uncommon event. These types of lesions respond well to treatment with steroids and 5-fluorouracil.[12,17]

Vascular compromise can occur when product is inadvertently injected into a blood vessel. This can cause ischemia with subsequent necrosis with or without scarring of the skin and soft tissue. Rarely, intravascular injections have led to occlusion of the ophthalmic and central retinal artery and blindness.[18]

Current recommendations to decrease the incidence of vascular events include low-pressure

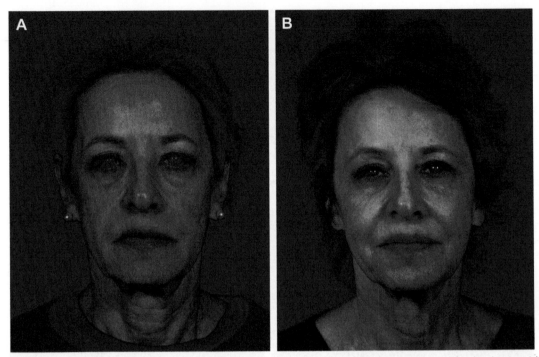

Fig. 9. A 68-year-old white woman seen before (*A*) and 1 year after (*B*) 8 sessions with 2 vials of poly-L-lactic acid/session done 6 months apart over the last 4 years. This patient had moderate to severe volume changes secondary to aging at the beginning of the treatment, and after discussion, elected to address this slowly over time with a product with long duration. She is satisfied with the result.

injections with small amounts of product through a constantly moving needle or cannula. This may serve to minimize both the number of events as well as the severity of an event should one occur. Extra care should be taken in areas with named vessels. Be aware that creases form over arterial vasculature and can provide us with a superficial topographic marker for their location.[19] A reflux maneuver (aspiration before injection) may reveal inadvertent intravascular placement of the needle before injection of product. This can be done with PLLA because it is a low-viscosity suspension injected with a fairly large (25 or 26) gauge needle. This is not possible with a thick product like Radiesse in a small syringe. Cannulas may be used, but be aware that these instruments can pierce and enter a vessel if force is applied, especially with the smaller cannulas.

If blanching is seen, the injection should be stopped immediately. The blanching is slowly replaced by a dusky reticulated pattern on the skin with slow capillary refill representing ischemia. Ischemia is painful (although lidocaine in the product may transiently prevent this) and depending on the extent of the injury may lead to necrosis of overlying tissue. Anticoagulation with aspirin, as well as heat and massage may help. The utility of nitroglycerin has recently been disputed.[20]

If an occlusion has occurred, but no blanching is seen, the patient may not call for hours, or even the next day, to complain of a purple area with or without pain. It is a good idea to make sure your front office staff are trained to have these patients come in to rule out occlusion as soon as possible (rather than dismiss it as a bruise). As these agents are not reversible, hyperbaric oxygen treatment to minimize tissue loss can be considered, and the earlier treatment is started the better.

POSTPROCEDURAL CARE/REHABILITATION AND RECOVERY

Postprocedural care is fairly similar after any injectable filler. The patient should avoid any vigorous exercise for a day or two to minimize swelling and erythema. If they experience mild pain, we recommend acetaminophen or nonsteroidal antiinflammatory drugs. As mentioned earlier, patients should be forewarned that they may swell a good deal after injections of Radiesse, but this will resolve in a couple of days. after treatment with PLLA, we recommend the patient massage the treated areas five times a day for 5 minutes for 5 days (rule of fives). This helps to increase the circulation in the treated areas.

SUMMARY

The demand for injectable fillers continues to increase year after year. For many patients, PLLA and CaHA provide an excellent treatment choice. Panfacial treatment with PLLA offers gradual, natural, and long-lasting results. It is also an excellent agent for treating lines in the décolleté area. Radiesse can be used along the jawline or as an injectable cheek or chin implant. In addition, it is a great product for the dorsal hands. With more refined technique and precise anatomically based treatment plans, a result can be achieved that meets or surpasses both patient and physician expectations. Complications are rare but do exist and anyone who plans to use the products must be knowledgeable of them and their management should they arise.

SUPPLEMENTARY DATA

Supplementary data related to this article can be found online at http://dx.doi.org/10.1016/j.fsc.2015.07.007.

REFERENCES

1. Gierloff M, Stöhring C, Buder T, et al. Aging changes of the midfacial fat compartments: a computed tomographic study. Plast Reconstr Surg 2012; 129(1):263–73.
2. Mendelson B, Wong C. Changes in the facial skeleton with aging: implications and clinical applications in facial rejuvenation. Aesthetic Plast Surg 2012;36:753–60.
3. Alghoul M, Codner M. Retaining ligaments of the face: review of anatomy and clinical applications. Aesthet Surg J 2013;33:769–82.
4. Attenello NH, Maas CS. Injectable fillers: review of material and properties. Facial Plast Surg 2015; 31(1):29–34.
5. ASPS Statistics. Available at: http://www.surgery.org/sites/default/files/2014-Stats.pdf. Accessed May 6, 2015.
6. Flaharty P. Radiance. Facial Plast Surg 2004;20(2): 165–9.
7. Berlin AL, Hussain M, Goldberg DJ. Calcium hydoxylapatite filler for facial rejuvenation: a histologic and immunohistochemical analysis. Dermatol Surg 2008; 34(Suppl 1):S64–7.
8. Sundaram H, Voigts B, Beer K, et al. Comparison of the rheological properties of viscosity and elasticity in two categories of soft tissue fillers: calcium hydroxylapatite and hyaluronic acid. Dermatol Surg 2010;36(Suppl 3):1859–65.
9. Fabi SG, Goldman MP. Hand rejuvenation: a review and our experience. Dermatol Surg 2012;38(7 Pt 2): 1112–27.
10. Vleggaar D. Facial volumetric correction with injectable poly-l-lactic acid. Dermatol Surg 2005;31: 1511–7.
11. Williams DF. On the mechanisms of biocompatibility. Biomaterials 2008;29:2941–53.
12. Fitzgerald R, Vleggaar D. Facial volume restoration of the aging face with poly-l-lactic acid. Dermatol Ther 2011;24:2–27.
13. Alessio R, Rzany B, Eve L, et al. European expert recommendations on the use of injectable poly-L-lactic acid for facial rejuvenation. J Drugs Dermatol 2014;13(9):1057–66.
14. Vleggaar D, Fitzgerald R, Lorenc ZP, et al. Consensus recommendations on the use of injectable poly-L-lactic acid for facial and nonfacial volumization. J Drugs Dermatol 2014;13(4 Suppl): s44–51.
15. Narins RS, Baumann L, Brandt FS, et al. a randomized study of the efficacy and safety of injectable poly-L-lactic acid versus human-based collagen implant in the treatment of nasolabial fold wrinkles. J Am Acad Dermatol 2010;62(3):448–62.
16. Vleggaar D, Fitzgerald R, Lorenc ZP. Understanding, avoiding, and treating potential adverse events following the use of injectable poly-L-lactic acid for facial and nonfacial volumization. J Drugs Dermatol 2014;13(4 Suppl):s35–9.
17. Bolton J, Fabi SG, Peterson J, et al. Poly-L-lactic acid for chest rejuvenation: a retrospective study of 28 cases using a 5-point chest wrinkle scale. Cosmet Dermatol 2011;24:278–84.
18. Lazzeri D, Agostini T, Figus M, et al. Blindness following cosmetic injections of the face. Plast Reconstr Surg 2012;129:995.
19. Pessa JE, Rohrich RJ. Facial topography clinical anatomy of the face. St Louis (MO): Quality Medical Publishing; 2012. p. 36–40.
20. Hwang CJ, Morgan PV, Pimentel A, et al. Rethinking the role of nitroglycerin ointment in ischemic vascular filler complications: an animal model. Ophthal Plast Reconstr Surg 2015. [Epub ahead of print].

Customized Approach to Facial Enhancement

Ava Shamban, MD*

KEYWORDS

• Precision • Injection • Midface • Volume • Lip structure • Anatomy

KEY POINTS

- The forehead ages in a similar fashion to the rest of the face with loss of volume in both subcutaneous fat and bone.
- Different injection techniques are recommended for the forehead, midface, lip, and lower face.
- From an aesthetic standpoint the entire perioral area must be treated, meaning the cutaneous lip, as well as the commissures and the chin.

INTRODUCTION

In recent years, there have been significant advances in understanding the anatomy and physiology of the aging face.[1-3] Although we understand the changes associated with aging from a global perspective, each individual ages at his or her own pace and in consideration to their specific anatomy.

For example, patients of Asian, Caucasian, Hispanic, and African descent demonstrate different changes in their anatomy as they age. When seen in the context of cumulative photodamage, some individuals see more descent and a thickening of their skin whereas others have more wrinkling and less descent. The overall shrinkage of the face that begins at the skeletal level extending to the superficial and deep fat pads and the skin envelope leads to unique alterations in the overall facial physiognomy. To provide optimal corrections to aging changes in the face, it behooves the treating physician to design an injection approach that addresses each individual based on their unique needs.

Evaluating the face in both a 2-dimensional and a 3-dimensional fashion is achieved using a combination of 3-dimensional imagery and calipers measuring the anatomic landmarks, such as the projection of the chin, the nose, the cheek, and the brow. The simplest clinical approach is to begin by dividing the face into thirds. The top third begins at the inferior aspect of the hairline, ending at the brow; the middle third begins at the brow and ends at the upper lip, and the lower third begins at the upper lip and ends at the chin and jaw line. This author likes to begin the process by first assessing the face as a single cosmetic unit and second, divide into thirds, and finally to use the phi principal of beauty to precisely determine how injections will ultimately deliver the optimal results in terms of reversal of aging and creating the most beautiful version of the person.[4,5]

ASSESSMENT AND TREATMENT OF THE TOP THIRD OF THE FACE

In a similar process to the entire face, the forehead flattens owing to loss of volume in both subcutaneous fat and bone. This leads to a skeletal appearance with flattening of the normal, pleasant youthful curve of the forehead, as well as prominence of veins that had not been visible in a younger face. The muscle responsible for lifting the brow and creating transverse wrinkles is the frontalis muscle, and in some individuals this motion creates deep horizontal lines in their forehead, **Fig. 1**.[6-8] Using newer techniques it is possible to safely revolumize the forehead in a judicial fashion.

AVA MD Santa Monica – Medical & Cosmetic Dermatology, 2021 Santa Monica Boulevard, Suite 600E, Santa Monica, CA 90404, USA
* AVA MD Beverly Hills – Medical & Cosmetic Dermatology, 9915 S. Santa Monica Boulevard, Beverly Hills, CA, 90212.
E-mail address: ava@avamd.com

Facial Plast Surg Clin N Am 23 (2015) 471–477
http://dx.doi.org/10.1016/j.fsc.2015.07.008
1064-7406/15/$ – see front matter © 2015 Elsevier Inc. All rights reserved.

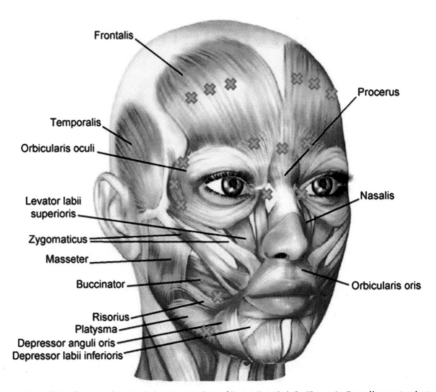

Fig. 1. The muscles of the face and toxin injection points. (*From* Bostini G, Figus A. Botulinum toxin type a treatment in facial rejuvenation. In: Giuseppe C, Antonio R, editors. Minimally invasive procedures for facial rejuvenation. Foster City (CA): OMICS Group; 2014. p. 11.)

One technique is to use a hyaluronic acid product such as Juvéderm Ultra, Restylane, or Boletero blended with one-third volume of plain lidocaine. This mixture allows for easier spread when injected into the subgaleal/periosteal plane. This author prefers to use a BD needle with a 0.30 mL syringe allowing precision injecting of small, controlled boluses of material. One can inject 0.05 to 0.10 mL at different points in the central forehead, well above the glabellar region, and gently spread the material using massage. This maneuver reestablishes the youthful curvature and softness seen in a younger face. Another technique is to use a cannula to deposit the filler in the subgaleal plane along with massage. This author has found this procedure to be more difficult in this area. Revolumizing the medial brow is necessary to lift the brow and soften the horizontal lines of the forehead, and returns the forehead to a more youthful look.[7]

Often, there is brow ptosis that occurs over time, owing to both bony loss, descent, and shrinkage of the underlying fat pad in the brow area. To reestablish the lift of the lateral brow, a combination approach using a neuromodulator such as, onabotulinumtoxinA, abobotulinumtoxinA or,

incobotulinumtoxinA, along with a hyaluronic acid is used. To lift the lateral brow, first assess the glabellar muscular complex and the orbicularis oculi to determine how many units of toxin are required to relax this depressor complex and the type of frown that the patient makes.[7,9,10] Then at the same time, or preferably at a second visit, the lateral brow can be injected, at the hairline just anterior or superior to the temporalis muscle, using anywhere from a 0.5 to 1 mL of either Restylane or Perlane because these agents are both slightly stiffer and provide more lift. In the temple, a blend of either 1.0 mL Juvéderm Ultra Plus or Perlane with 0.5 mL plain lidocaine is injected down to periosteum. For the lateral tail of the brow, injecting just underneath the dermis and into the subcutaneous fat pad using anywhere from 0.1 or 0.2 mL Juvéderm Ultra or Restylane, not blended so as to avoid diffusion of the product. Another nice technique is to use a cannula in the subcutaneous space beneath the tail of the brow.

The author recommends a judicial use of neurotoxin in the upper third of the face. The muscular complex that forms the glabellar region including the corrugators, procerus, and parts of the orbicularis oculi can be treated in a relatively low-dose fashion to avoid a frozen look. This author recommends evaluating the musculature to determine the number of units necessary to achieve a relaxed look.

For the brow area, once again the author recommends a more conservative approach to neurotoxin dosing to allow for more movement of the forehead. In the crow's feet area, because the orbicularis oculi is very thin, this author treats where the patients muscle is contracting and use anywhere from 6 to 12 U.[11]

ASSESSMENT AND TREATMENT OF THE MIDFACE

There has been an enormous step forward in the assessment and treatment of the midface.[12] We now understand how the treatment of the midface impacts both the nasolabial fold and the commissures. Accurate treatment can deliver on the promise of beautifying the face by establishing a stronger projection of the malar eminence, maxilla, and curve of the cheek.[13] With appropriate distribution of volume of product the skin envelope will redrape. In general, product placement is planned using Hinderer's lines (Fig. 2). The injection begins from the superior point of the malar eminence continuing onto the inferior maxillary zone.[14] Injecting directly on top of the periosteum

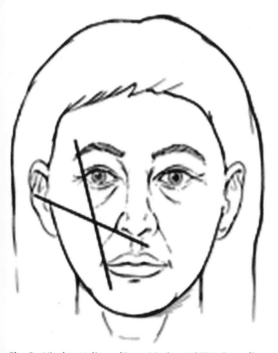

Fig. 2. Hinderer's lines. (*From* Marianetti TM, Cozzolino S, Torroni A, et al. The "beauty arch:" a new aesthetic analysis for malar augmentation planning. J Craniofac Surg 2015;26(3):627; with permission.)

lifts up the superficial and deep fat pads. Injections are continued medially, as described by Montes[13] and they define the midface and lower jawline.

For the midface, it is important to use a product that has a higher G prime, such as Voluma, Perlane, or Radiesse.[4] The technique that this author uses is to deliver boluses of 0.20 mL spaced about 2 cm apart in the areas that have been described by Swift and Remington.[5] The deeper plane injections will redrape the skin by suspending the skin between pillars, in the same fashion that a tent pole holds up a tent. For example, a very straightforward and predictable treatment approach is injecting 0.20 mL in A1 and A2, and then 0.10 mL in A3 on both sides of the face.

The underlying cause of the nasolabial fold is often the descent of the malar fat pad. Because this has been addressed by treatment of the midface the nasolabial fold is evaluated after the midcheek has been treated. In prior years, the nasolabial fold was overtreated giving patients a snoutlike appearance. If there is a residual nasolabial fold after the treatment of the midface, this author prefers to use a mattressing or fern technique, where the product is injected from the cheek down to the base of the nose and then continuing perpendicular to the line, all the way to the lateral oral commissure. This sequence tends to give a better lift to the nasolabial fold when it is severe.[15] In elderly patients this may be the only way to soften the nasolabial fold. If there is a wrinkle on top of the nasolabial fold, the area is retreated 2 weeks later by injecting a filler at a superficial level, either dermal or subdermal plane, using either Boletero, Restylane, or Juvéderm.

ASSESSMENT AND TREATMENT OF THE LOWER FACE: LIPS, CHIN, AND JAWLINE

The lower third of the face includes the oral commissures, marionette lines, chin, jaw line, and the perioral area including the lips. As in other areas of the face, combining a sharp needle, cannula, blended, and nonblended hyaluronic acid or calcium hydroxyapatite is recommended as a general rule.

To address the marionette lines, filler is injected beginning at the jaw line and advancing up to the oral commissures using a pillar technique (see Figs. 4 and 5). The product is injected in 0.10- to 0.20-mL aliquots at a 90° angle to the skin similar to laying down a pillar that, in effect, lifts the skin up, and in turn lifts the entire area. Neurotoxin is injected at the insertion of the depressor angular oris muscle at the mandible. This improves allows full correction of the marionette line.[11,16]

To address the oral commissure, this author often loads the product into a 0.30-mL BD syringe and injects lateral to the oral commissure, beginning at the modiolus advancing toward the angle of the mouth. The objective is to create a neutral commissure, neither angling up into a jokerlike appearance nor drooping down giving a sad appearance.

Along with the eyes, the lips form the central feature of the face. It is an area that is often over-injected or completely ignored. In either situation, not treating this area can destroy the overall look of the face. From an aesthetic standpoint, the entire perioral area must be treated, meaning the cutaneous lip, as well as the commissures and the chin. Hyaluronic acid–based dermal fillers are commonly used for aesthetic lip augmentation procedures to increase lip fullness, define the lips, and restore perioral volume loss that may occur with aging and actinic damage.[17] To achieve the goal of an aesthetically pleasing lip, it is important to evaluate each individual's lip structure (**Fig. 3**).[18] Depending on ethnicity, the ratio of the lower lip to the upper lip should be 1.5:1 ratio, except in patients of African or Asian ethnicity, where the lips may be 1:1 ratio. In addition, the shape of the lip can vary dramatically between individuals and ethnicities. Some individuals have a more prominent cupid's bow, almost a V-shape, other patients will have a softer rounder cupid's bow, whereas others still have no cupids bow and only have a soft arch to their upper lip.

The clinician must take into consideration the shape and size of the lip, because that will determine the quantity used there. Whatever the injection technique, care should be taken to inject an amount of filler in a given location sufficient to achieve lip correction without distorting the natural anatomy orientation of the lips.[17]

To address the lip, this author always begins with the perioral area. In a younger face, the perioral area may be completely intact, that is, without wrinkles and require no additional volume. Only an enhancement of the aesthetic shape of the lip or a small amount of volume may be needed to create an attractive pout or appearance of the lower lip. Alternatively, the upper lip may be too small for the dentition or for the face. In a more mature face, the entire perioral area often needs volume to eliminate deeper lines, hide visible veins, and address the entire shrunken perioral area both above and below the lip. It is very easy to revolumize this area with a fairly small amount of product. This author often blends Juvéderm Ultra Plus or Restylane and inject anywhere from 0.50 to 1.0 mL across the entire perioral area, both above and below the lip, using either a needle in a linear retrograde threading technique or with a 27-gauge cannula. After the perioral area is filled, the anatomic landmarks of the lip are then reestablished.

This author always initiates lip restoration in the upper lip by outlining the cupids bow. Using a 0.3-mL BD syringe, the injection begins at the lateral commissure using 0.05 to 0.10 mL of Restylane or Juvéderm. These products both can define the arch of the bow by creating a white roll and a slight eversion of the lip eliminating any lines that begin in the white lip continuing down to the pink lip (**Figs. 4–7**). The second step is to add a small amount of volume, either Restylane Silk, Restylane, or Juvederm, to the body of the lip, just above the wet/dry border, usually 0.1 to 0.2 mL per side.[19] Finally, the author augments the cupid's peak with

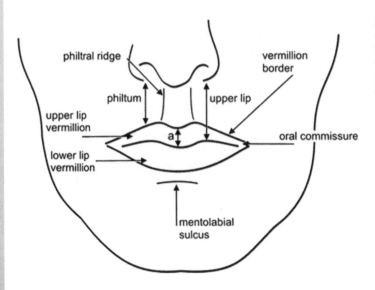

Fig. 3. Diagram of the lip. (*From* Carey JC, Cohen MM, Curry CJ, et al. Elements of morphology: standard terminology for the lips, mouth, and oral region. Am J Med Genet A 2009;149(1):78; with permission.)

philtral ridge

vermillion border

philtrum

upper lip

upper lip vermillion

a

oral commissure

lower lip vermillion

mentolabial sulcus

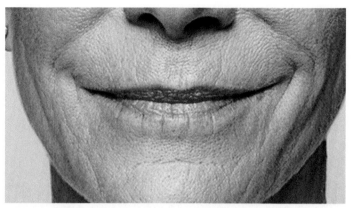

Fig. 4. Patient before lip injections and perioral injections of hyaluronic acid.

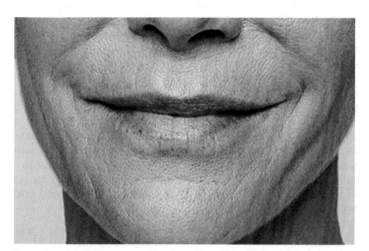

Fig. 5. Patient after lip and perioral injections of hyaluronic acid.

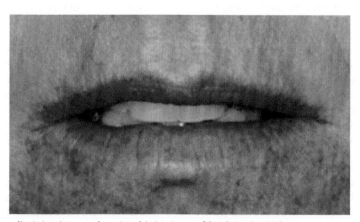

Fig. 6. Patient before lip injections and perioral injections of hyaluronic acid.

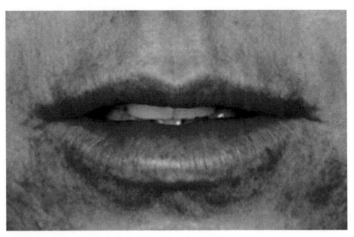

Fig. 7. Patient after lip and perioral injections of hyaluronic acid.

0.05 mL to each peak. Reestablishing the philtral columns is necessary both to eliminate any horizontal lines below the columella and to shorten the cutaneous lip. It requires 0.05 or 0.1 mL per column creating an A-line, not an H appearance.

Treating the chin can give a pleasing profile in general to the face and also serve to tighten up the lax skin along the jawline. The chin can be injected both above the muscle and directly on the periosteum to rebuild the bony structure, as well as provide structure and volume to the skin. The product, which can either be a hyaluronic acid or calcium hydroxyapatite, can be injected directly onto the periosteum at a 90° angle at the base of the chin, after withdrawing the syringe to make certain there is no inadvertent entry into a blood vessel. The author uses several injection points using a sharp needle, delivering 0.20 mL and covering the entire projection of the chin, using only about 0.50 to 1.0 mL in total. Finally, the author injects in the subdermal plane above the muscle using anywhere from 0.25 to 1.0 mL. The chin is gently molded with massage using ultrasound gel.

The jawline can be treated in linear fashion using a combination of sharp needle and a 25-gauge cannula. First, boluses of 0.1 or 0.2 mL are placed at the posterior ramus, along the curve of the ramus and at the chin. These injections serve to stretch the skin, giving a nice lift and definition to the jaw line as well as picking up the upper third of the neck. Using a cannula, placing threads of either a hyaluronic acid or calcium hydroxyapatite along the ramus provides definition to the jawline. The author also use a neuromodulator to accomplish the so-called Nefertiti neck lift along the jawline.[20] This technique relaxes the top part of the platysma, adding to the definition of the jaw line. The platysma bands can be treated simultaneously to relax their downward pull, also giving emphasis and lift to the jawline.

SUMMARY

Creating a refreshed, best version of an individual face requires knowledge of facial anatomy, understanding of the interactions of fillers and neurotoxins with tissue and muscle, and dedication to the primary principal of aesthetic responsibility. As physicians, we know to "do no harm" and when it comes to aesthetics, this author believes it is our responsibility to create beauty and not distortion.

REFERENCES

1. Bartus CL, Sattler G, Hanke CW. The tower technique: a novel technique for the injection of hyaluronic acid fillers. J Drugs Dermatol 2011;10(11):1277–80.
2. Coleman SR, Grover R. The anatomy of the aging face: volume loss and changes in 3-dimensional topography. Aesthet Surg J 2006;26(1S):S4–9.
3. Rohrich RJ, Pessa JE. The fat compartments of the face: anatomy and clinical implications for cosmetic surgery. Plast Reconstr Surg 2007;119(7):2219–27.
4. Muhn C, Rosen N, Solish N, et al. The evolving role of hyaluronic acid fillers for facial volume restoration and contouring: a Canadian overview. Clin Cosmet Investig Dermatol 2012;5:147–58.
5. Swift A, Remington K. BeautiPHIcation™: a global approach to facial beauty. Clin Plast Surg 2011; 38(3):347–77.
6. Bostini G, Figus A. Botulinum toxin type a treatment in facial rejuvenation. In: Giuseppe C, Antonio R, editors. Minimally invasive procedures for facial rejuvenation. Foster City (CA): OMICS Group; 2014. p. 1–42.

7. Nanda S, Bansal S. Upper face rejuvenation using botulinum toxin and hyaluronic acid fillers. Indian J Dermatol Venereol Leprol 2013;79(1):32–40.

8. Redbord K, Pagliai KP. Soft-tissue augmentation with hyaluronic acid and calcium hydroxyl apatite fillers. Dermatol Ther 2011;24(1):71.

9. Carruthers JD, Glogau RG, Blitzer A, Facial Aesthetics Consensus Group Faculty. Advances in facial rejuvenation: botulinum toxin type a, hyaluronic acid dermal fillers, and combination therapies-consensus recommendations. Plast Reconstr Surg 2008; 121(Suppl 5):5S–30S [quiz: 31S–6S].

10. de Maio M. Treatment planning. Injectable fillers in aesthetic medicine. Foster City (CA): Springer; 2014. p. 41–59.

11. Wollina U. Perioral rejuvenation: restoration of attractiveness in aging females by minimally invasive procedures. Clin Interv Aging 2013;8:1149.

12. Hoffmann K, Juvéderm Voluma Study Investigators Group. Volumizing effects of a smooth, highly cohesive, viscous 20-mg/mL hyaluronic acid volumizing filler: prospective European study. BMC Dermatol 2009;9(9):1–9.

13. Montes JR. Volumetric considerations for lower eyelid and midface rejuvenation. Curr Opin Ophthalmol 2012;23(5):443–9.

14. Marianetti TM, Cozzolino S, Torroni A, et al. The "beauty arch:" a new aesthetic analysis for malar augmentation planning. J Craniofac Surg 2015;26(3):625–30.

15. Weinkle SH and Maher IA. Melomental folds. In: Soft tissue augmentation: procedures in cosmetic dermatology series. Elsevier; 2012. p. 147.

16. Belmontesi M, Grover R, Verpaele A. Transdermal injection of Restylane SubQ for aesthetic contouring of the cheeks, chin, and mandible. Aesthet Surg J 2006;26(1 Suppl):S28–34.

17. Smith SR, Lin X, Shamban A. Small gel particle hyaluronic acid injection technique for lip augmentation. J Drugs Dermatol 2013;12(7):764–9.

18. Carey JC, Cohen MM, Curry CJ, et al. Elements of morphology: standard terminology for the lips, mouth, and oral region. Am J Med Genet A 2009; 149(1):77–92.

19. Glogau RG, Bank D, Brandt F, et al. A Randomized, evaluator-blinded, controlled study of the effectiveness and safety of small gel particle hyaluronic acid for lip augmentation. Dermatol Surg 2012;38: 1180–92.

20. Joseph JH. Nonsurgical neck laxity correction. Clin Plast Surg 2014;41(1):7–9.

Injectable Filler Techniques for Facial Rejuvenation, Volumization, and Augmentation

Lawrence S. Bass, MD, FACS

KEYWORDS

- Hyaluronic acid • Calcium hydroxylapatite • Augmentation • Injectable • Filler • Facial

KEY POINTS

- Fillers are selected based on the biophysical properties for the tissue depth and type of correction contemplated.
- Fillers can restore facial volume aging loss or change the shape of the face.
- A combination of injection techniques usually produces a more complete correction.
- Correction of all of the deficits in a given region produces a more complete and harmonious correction than treating isolated features.

INTRODUCTION

Injectable fillers have become a prominent part of modern facial rejuvenation with more than 1.9 million treatments a year in the United States.[1] This growing popularity has been fueled by the advent of multiple biocompatible and reasonably durable filler materials, most notably hyaluronic acid (HA) fillers, allowing a number of previously unmet needs to be addressed in a predictable and reproducible manner. Treatment of facial volume loss owing to aging is the most common application, correcting a variety of early and late changes. The immediacy, predictability, and safety of these no-downtime treatments make them the treatment of choice in most clinical circumstances. By adding volume or shape restoration of the aging face, in combination with energy-based treatments (lasers, radiofrequency, and others) for skin surface changes, such as wrinkles and pigmentary changes, and surgical lifting for skin laxity, a more complete correction of the aging face can be obtained.

GENERAL APPROACH

Detailed knowledge of facial anatomy, typical aging changes in the face, and aesthetic planning are essential to obtain artistic, balanced, natural-looking results. Filler injection is extremely technique dependent. Basically, a 3-dimensional latticework of injected material is being placed beneath the skin surface to add volume, change surface conformation, or thicken skin or subcutaneous tissues or fill a rhytid. All of these things are a form of sculpture, which result in a change in facial appearance. The degree of correction and the volume required for any given result is greatly dependent on the injection technique used. Likewise, pushing beyond the limits of what the treatments can reasonably produce is a sure recipe for unnatural looking results, or worse, tissue damage and complications. As benign as these treatments are in most cases, even after repetitive treatments, excessive volume or frequency of treatment is likely to result in trouble that is otherwise easily avoided.

Disclosures: Advisory Boards, Allergan, Merz.
Bass Plastic Surgery, PLCC, 568 Park Avenue, New York, NY 10065, USA
E-mail address: drbass@drbass.net

Facial Plast Surg Clin N Am 23 (2015) 479–488
http://dx.doi.org/10.1016/j.fsc.2015.07.004

There are many specific details to treating each anatomic area of the face. However, there are certain overall principles that apply in all these areas. First, no one filler is the correct choice for any application. Next, no one filler is going to be optimal for all the application areas in routine clinical practice. Each provider must select at least a small number of fillers to stock and needs to become facile at the specific feel and nuances of those fillers.

CHOICE OF FILLER

As stated, no one filler is the correct choice for any application. Like selecting a golf club for a particular shot, a few clubs may be workable in skillful hands. Clearly, some choices will not work in a given situation (eg, a very soft, spreadable filler will not create a sharp, sculpted shape in the cheeks). The starting place for filler selection in this author's hands relates to the anticipated depth of placement. Subcutaneous or supraperiosteal (but an exception is in the orbital area) fillers are generally heavier, which means higher viscosity and cohesivity. Fillers such as calcium hydroxylapatite (CaHa) and high-viscosity, high-cohesivity HA fall into this category. The original lower viscosity HA fillers work well in the deep dermal tissue plane or at the dermal/subcutaneous junction. Thinner fillers (which have lower viscosity and elastic modulus) such as monophasic, polydensified HA are suitable for middermal injection. The circumstances most appropriate for a given depth of injection are illustrated in detail in the specific anatomic application areas discussed elsewhere in this article.

At the time of this writing, the filler selection approved by the US Food and Drug Administration (FDA) for aesthetic use is a relatively short list. With the introduction of multiple new fillers to the marketplace, filler selection will necessarily change. Such selection is guided by the general principles discussed herein, clinical experience, and performance of the new product as determined by the community of clinical providers after several years of use and the filler alternatives available at that particular time. The techniques and selection presented herein represent this author's preferred or usual techniques, but certainly not the only or necessarily best option. Each physician must base clinical choices on what works best in his or her hands.

Although neocollagenesis secondary to a pressure phenomenon inducing collagen synthesis in fibroblasts has been demonstrated secondary to HA filler injection, the magnitude of collagen replacement attributable to this mechanism is unclear.[2] Nonetheless, recurrent treatment with HA fillers seems to provide longer intervals and reduced volumes after several treatments, suggesting that there is clinical significance to these findings.

It is not necessary to stock all HA fillers. Wide cross-applicability exists; however, this author believes that the fine features of each filler provide nuance to the correction that make them preferable for certain treatments. Other injectors might prefer a different filler.

CaHa particles stimulate neocollagenesis through an inflammatory-mediated mechanism that produces significant collagen to replace the gel carrier which absorbs over the first 3 to 4 months. This is a unique combination of time zero contour improvement followed by neocollagenesis. The filler also has mechanical properties that are unique, providing a high elastic modulus compared with other available products. The safety profile and tolerance of the material is excellent even after recurrent use of significant volumes.[3] Owing to the time zero correction, a close match between what you see during treatment and what you get in clinical correction—stiffer mechanical properties and greater longevity—this filler is well-suited where defined shapes or sculpting are needed.

This author has restricted clinical practice to using only biological fillers with FDA approval for an aesthetic facial indication. Nonbiological, nonabsorbable materials in soft tissue locations have had a troubled past. Owing to the permanent nature of many of these materials, the potential for late misadventure is concerning. Breakdown of the materials after protracted residence in the body is another issue that will only manifest many years after adoption of a new material. Concern regarding biofilm formation on such materials is also a factor. Given the appropriately low tolerance of providers and patients for complications with aesthetic treatments, the biological, absorbable options seem preferable, particularly given the increased filler volumes and treatment frequencies that are being used. Whether a nonbiological nonabsorbable filler that is biocompatible and safe over the long term will be developed in the near future remains to be seen.

Because the details of differences in crosslinking and physical structure between different HA fillers is discussed elsewhere in this volume, this article does not reiterate these facts, but summarizes by saying that these differences affect physical properties, which in turn affect the clinical performance of the fillers.[4] Clearly, as more fillers enter the marketplace, a careful understanding of multiple physical properties of the fillers is going to be increasingly important to aid in filler selection.

The details presented herein represent this author's preferred injection techniques as a snapshot at the time of this writing. Other injection techniques might perform just as well and different techniques might be useful in an individual patient. The introduction of new fillers will change this perspective continuously, both in terms of inclusion of new filler options and the optimal techniques for injecting them.

FACIAL REJUVENATION WITH FILLERS: VOLUME RESTORATION

Volume restoration of the aging face has become the most commonplace mainstay of medical facial rejuvenation. The face begins losing fat start some time in the late 30s. This produces a change in facial shape with blunting of the prominence and width of the malar eminence, loss of definition of the angle of the jaw, and descent of the cheek fat pads. Not only is the face losing fat, but fat pads in the face are either descending and/or losing volume at different rates, creating visible segmenting of facial compartments that seemed to be confluent in youth.[5] These changes, along with loss of skin elasticity and development of skin laxity, result in progressive deepening of folds and creases in the face. The primary treatment for such changes, particularly early in the aging process, is with injectable fillers.

LIQUID FACELIFT: THE ROLE OF VOLUMIZATION IN SKIN LAXITY

With a patient population that is increasingly averse to operative procedures and anxious to minimize or even avoid recovery time, providers have added volume in the form of off-the-shelf fillers to take up some of the slack in lax facial skin. This is particularly helpful in the cheek, jowl, and nasolabial areas and to some extent in the brow and upper eyelid. The neck is not amenable to a decrease in laxity using injectable fillers. Because the face loses volume during aging, some measure of volume restoration has a good biological rationale, in addition to the practical dimension. For early facial aging, or a small degree of contour improvement, injectable fillers work quite well. Fat grafting is an alternative, albeit one with a trip to the operating room and at least some recovery time.

For patients with moderate or advanced skin laxity, fillers do not provide a meaningful option because the amount of volume required is both cost prohibitive and will leave the patient looking overplumped which is not a desirable aesthetic enhancement, even if less skin laxity is apparent. As in all treatment decision making, staying within the boundaries of a natural appearance shows us where to draw the line and move on to a bigger intervention, like surgical lifting.

CHANGING FACIAL FEATURES WITH FILLER

Many facial features can be altered modestly to moderately using injectable fillers in either the aging patient or the youthful patient. Filler injections in the cheeks, chin, nose, brows, and angle of the jaw can create a change in facial shape separate from restoration of youthful appearance. This technique has the advantage of adjustability in very small increments to create small changes that can not be produced reliably using surgical techniques. Often, patients who are actors, models, or in similar careers need very small shape adjustments to improve symmetry or refine the details of their appearance. Substantial changes are best addressed with solid facial implants or osteotomies. Fillers also have a role in camouflaging the visible edge of an implant, especially in the very thin patient or the patient with a very large implant.

NASOLABIAL FOLD

This treatment area, which represented the test bed for most of the studies of FDA-approved fillers, remains a mainstay of clinical treatment. Although it has fallen into disfavor with some, because it is not a prominent aging feature or is better corrected with filler cheek augmentation, it is included in most of this author's treatment planning for naïve or relatively inexperienced patients. Patients in their late 30s and early 40s or beyond almost always benefit from a modest appropriate amount of correction of the nasolabial fold.

The depth increases with aging in most patients, but other features need to be assessed during treatment planning. Asymmetries need to be assessed and demonstrated to the patient before treatment. These asymmetries will be blunted by filler augmentation, but rarely completely eliminated. The degree of depth correction needs to be modest and natural looking. The nasolabial fold is a normal facial feature in youth and should not be completely effaced or bulging with convexity at any point.

In addition to nasolabial depth, the presence of any dermal rhytid along the length of the fold should be noted. In patients with a rhytid, this author selects an HA filler that can be placed both in the deep dermis or dermal subcutaneous junction as well as in the mid dermis for more complete correction of the rhytid as well as fold depth. Alternatively, CaHa can be selected for deep correction at the dermal subcutaneous junction followed by middermal correction of the rhytid. This bilayer treatment can be done in 1 sitting or in an alternating fashion. Patients need to be questioned about which feature of the fold they find most objectionable; some patients have a strong prioritization to focus on correction of the rhytid rather than the depth or the other way around.

The final assessment is the presence or absence and severity of overhanging inferomedial cheek skin, which will also modulate the injection technique. Severe skin overhang is best corrected with facialplasty or a middle facelift to resuspend the cheek. Moderate skin redundancy here ideally requires cross-hatching transversely across the fold to better flatten and structure the skin surface conformation, as well as some filler cheek augmentation. Mild redundancy is usually amenable to cross-hatching alone. The absence of any noticeable degree of skin redundancy is ideal for a fold-only volume fill with a fanning technique. Treatment can proceed without following this protocol, but the patient should be cautioned of this compromise and the resulting incomplete correction of overhanging skin.

For basic fold filling, a fanning technique is used, inserting the needle inferiorly on the fold and advancing it superiorly to the apex at the base of the nose (**Fig. 1**). Injection is made retrograde

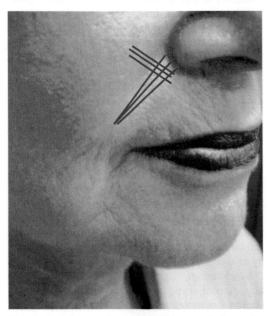

Fig. 1. Fanning and cross-hatching technique for correction of the nasolabial fold.

placing 0.05 to 0.1 mL of material in each pass until optimal correction is obtained. Both CaHa and HA work well in this area, preferably mixed with 0.2 to 0.3 mL of 1% lidocaine with epinephrine to help minimize ecchymosis. It is more difficult to produce an overfilled look or an unnatural surface feature with subdermal rather than intradermal placement of filler.

Residual depth at the superior portion of the fold can be further corrected using cross-hatching from a needle introduced lateral to the fold and advanced toward the midline. Retrograde injection is then made as the needle is withdrawn. This is also used for mild to moderate redundant cheek skin immediately above or lateral to the fold. Fill in the depth of the fold can be subcutaneous, but at the lateral edge of the fold and lateral to the fold the cross-hatched threads should be at the dermal subcutaneous junction or deep dermis and very thin. This lateral cross-hatching is intended to change the surface conformation of the skin, tenting it flatter.

MARIONETTE LINE

Unlike the nasolabial fold, which is present in youth, the marionette line is only a feature in the aging face. As such, complete effacement is desirable but is never achieved in practice. This is in part owing to the fibrous septae ("ligaments") dividing fat compartments in this part of the face, as well as to dermal attachments to muscular fascia. Nonetheless, significant improvement can be obtained. Surface creases in the oral commissure are best corrected using an HA filler that can be lined (threaded superficially—middermis) into the crease and then filler infiltrated in small amounts in the entire patch of skin in the corner of the mouth to structure or flatten these tissues. Some limitation in correction is inevitable owing to fibrous septae between the skin and deeper tissues, segmenting fat compartments in this area. Biplanar correction in the dermis and subcutaneously can provide a more complete correction.

Treatment in this area is highly individualized and based on the findings in each patient. Supporting the corners of the mouth, which progressively sink in and lose support, creating a frowning appearance, is almost always necessary (**Fig. 2**). Direct fill of the marionette line and some cross-hatching to structure this skin flat is also common. Variations may take account of contour depressions in the labiomental groove. Just lateral to this, a triangular depression is often seen, which was not present in youth or which has become more pronounced with aging. Fanning subcutaneously provides good correction of this feature.

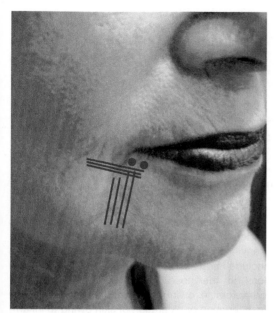

Fig. 2. Fanning and cross-hatching technique for correction of the marionette line area.

LIPS
Aging Restoration

May patients in the aging population are afraid to consider this correction owing to some of the overblown treatments they have seen in younger patients. Filler injection in the lip in aging patients is typically more focused on restoring or accenting the natural curves of the lip and reflating the lip to minimize vermillion creasing, along with correcting rhytids in the white lip skin. A thinner, flatter lip typically develops during aging, which blunts the natural curves of a youthful lip. Correction centers on accentuation of the natural curves of the lip, namely, the tubercle and cupids bow peaks in particular with minimal accent of the white roll if needed and desired by the patient. Vermillion is enhanced only to the extent needed to fill the deflated contour or only partially if full correction will be out of balance with the patient's other facial contours.

These changes are accomplished by injection in the white roll or vermillion–cutaneous junction, which should flow along the entire roll in the correct plane (**Fig. 3**). A small bleb of material at the cupid's bow peak itself with a somewhat stiffer HA accents this feature nicely. Occasionally, the philthral columns will also be minimally injected. Overinjection of the white roll produces an unnatural "duck bill" lip, which is a telltale of a treated lip. This can also be produced by very heavy augmentation of the vermillion, which pushes up the white roll.

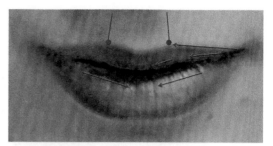

Fig. 3. Options for shaping the lip.

Vermillion corrections, including the tubercle, are made at the vermillion–mucosal junction in the submuscular plane with a small, secondary injection midway across the vermillion width if needed for more complete reflation. The youthful, beautiful vermillion shape is most commonly viewed as most prominent at the tubercle in the upper lip, with an adjacent area of relative emptiness and then relative fullness or convexity that tapers medial to lateral. The "puffy" lip, which is overfilled laterally, is another tell-tale of an unnatural treated lip. Similarly, the upper lip that is filled uniformly across its full length or across each side of the lip from commissure to tubercle is demonstrably unnatural. The border of the lip at the oral aperture should be ideally curved and not straight. This means that the level of fill needs to vary continuously across the lip to produce a natural shape.

Augmentation of the lips in younger patients follows the injection techniques described, but with greater volumes, particularly in the vermillion to enhance lip size and shape more noticeably. This should still be kept in proportion to the general facial features present rather than creating a lip or perioral contour that is outsized in comparison to the rest of the face.

PREJOWL SULCUS

As patients age, progressive descent and loss of fat pads in the face, combined with loss of skin elasticity, contribute to the formation of the jowl. As aging progresses, bone loss may also contribute to the appearance of a depression or mild notch between the jowl and bony mentum with overlying fat pad. Treatment of mild jowling involves injection of the prejowl sulcus to camouflage the depression between the jowl and mentum by creating a smooth ramp or graded transition between the 2 areas rather than a relative concavity or depression (**Fig. 4**). Moderate or worse jowl formation and laxity should be addressed more properly with surgical lifting, but can be somewhat minimized by filler injection as a compromise maneuver.

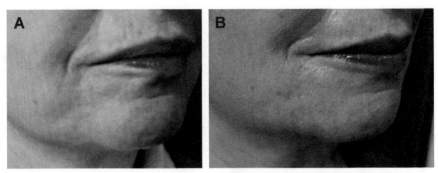

Fig. 4. (*A*) Early jowl before treatment. (*B*) After filler correction anterior to the jowl.

Multiple injection techniques are possible, including deep dermal or dermal–subcutaneous junction injection between the 2 areas using a fanning or cross-hatching technique for the approximate height of the visible jowl. Another technique places "pillars" of material in small bleb or bolus injections deep under the soft tissues supraperiosteally or in a deep to superficial column to raise the surface contour.

This author's preferred method of correction focuses on restoring the inferior border of the mandible between the 2 areas with subcutaneous injection in a linear threading fashion. If generalized depression is present in the area in more advanced aging changes, minimal threading or cross-hatching for the approximate vertical height of the jowl can be performed. The needle is inserted within the skin of the jowl and/or within the skin of the mentum and threaded into the prejowl sulcus along the inferior border of the mandible. Injection is made while withdrawing the needle to differentially build the surface contour to ramp smoothly from the jowl to chin. Care must be taken to avoid the facial artery and vein and their side branches, which can result in profound ecchymosis that can take 2 weeks or more to clear fully. Patients should be cautioned about increased risk of bruising in this area as with eyelid injections.

NOSE

Small shape changes in the dorsum or tip can be effected using injectable fillers. This is often useful in patients with aesthetic deformities too small to reliably refine with surgical correction or who will not consider surgical treatment. Trialing a possible surgical result or appearance can also allow some patients to proceed with more confidence to surgical correction, although no guarantee can be made that the same appearance can be produced surgically.

Although the virtues of nonoperative nasal shaping seem appealing, caution is in order. The nose is a highly vascular structure with thin tissues under some pressure and tension against the underlying osseocartilaginous framework. Risks include intravascular injection with possible tissue loss in the nose, stroke, blindness, vascular compromise owing to compression with tissue loss, erosion or ulceration of skin owing to inflammation, and induration or skin atrophy owing to inflammation or compression. These concerns are accentuated in the patient receiving multiple injections or with significant scar or vascular compromise from multiple previous nasal surgeries. The surgeon should be aware that subsequent surgery may pose more technical challenges and risks in the multiply injected patient.

Injection is made in the deep dermis or subcutaneously in the tip and subcutaneously in the dorsum. Small amounts should be used with short linear threads, avoiding the temptation to place significant boluses of material with the needle in a fixed position. Molding or rolling can be used minimally to smooth the injected material into the desired contour.

CHEEK COMPLEX

The cheek has several zones that are important to consider in aesthetic planning. Each of these zones may be deficient owing to aging changes with volume loss or descent. These changes progress at different rates in each fat pad, changing confluent shapes of youth into discontinues segments and changing the proportions of the face. Fibrous septae or "ligaments" between fat pads become visible as creases. Augmentation of this area is designed to restore the original volume and proportions with the lateral malar/zygomatic area showing as the widest portion of the face. Creases or depressions between fat pads need to be minimized. Beyond this, the region can be enhanced to create a more beautiful appearance than the patient had in youth—a more beautiful, normal by creating more definition and sculpting in this region. The same enhancement can be created as a mild or moderate cheek augmentation in the youthful patient. Injectable fillers have the advantage of finely gradable and customizable shapes and sizes in each part of the cheek compared with surgically placed cheek implants, with less durability as a disadvantage.

Areas to consider include lateral cheek (zygomaticomalar complex), medial cheek, submalar hollowing, and creases or depressions between fat pads of the cheek. In facial lipoatrophy, a depression superolateral to the nasolabial fold is a unique feature that needs to be addressed that is not usually seen in the aging face patient. In terms of aesthetic planning, this author feels that most patients benefit from enhancement of the lateral portion of the cheek including the malar complex and sweeping slightly superior and lateral to strengthen the width of the midface along with modest enhancement of the anterior projection. Except for addressing malar creasing, this author does not usually inject the medial portion of the cheek in most Caucasian aging patients because this author believes that the inferomedial portion of the cheek above the nasolabial fold becomes heavier and fuller. Aside from malar creases between fat pads or extending inferiorly from the tear trough, little volume is required in this area. However, many Asian patients or other patients with a broad, flat midfacial physiognomy may benefit aesthetically from enhancement to create fullness and convexity in this region.

Lateral areas are usually corrected with 1 to 2 boluses of material placed deep under the malar fat pad or supraperiosteal to lift and accent the most prominent portion of the malar eminence. CaHa or high-cohesivity HA fillers provide the rheological properties to create good lifting effects. The former can be molded easily into the final shape desired after injecting the bolus (es) including a final bolus along the zygomatic arch (**Fig. 5**). High-cohesivity HA does not mold as easily and is either injected in smaller boluses deep or in small columns or pillars injected retrograde while withdrawing the needle which, has been placed deep. This technique also works well for this material when injecting the creases compared with CaHa, which this author typically threads into creases. Overcorrection of the superior border of the malar area can accentuate the lid–cheek junction, however.

Submalar hollowing is a question of magnitude and moderation. A neutral or slightly concave contour is acceptable or even desirable but greater degrees of hollowing contribute to the gaunt, "worn-out" look of aging in both the cheek and temple areas. Submalar hollowing responds well to all manner of filler materials using a fanning or cross-hatched fanning approach subcutaneously. The goal is to moderate pronounced hollowing leaving the contour neutral or just concave. Convexity is undesirable, creating a chipmunk cheek appearance at worse or a baby face at best. If a very youthful baby face is the aesthetic desire of the patient, rounding the malar area rather than overprojecting the submalar area may be preferable.

JAWLINE

The jawline changes in many ways with aging. As in other areas of the face, these changes are products of soft tissue as well as bony changes. These areas typically become more prominent at different decades in the aging process. Correct balance or restoration of the youthful shape as verified by old photographs of the patient aged 30s help to get it right. Overwidening the jaw to

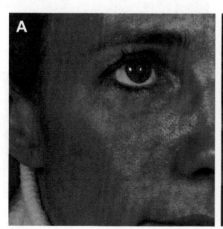 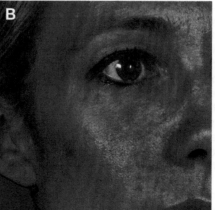

Fig. 5. (*A*) Before treatment. (*B*) After filler augmentation of the cheek.

accommodate skin laxity can produce a grotesque, outsized face that looks particularly unflattering in women.

After the prejowl sulcus, which is discussed elsewhere in this article, the mandibular angle is the next most commonly corrected jawline shape. Soft tissue loss and migration over the angle produces diminished facial width in this area. In conjunction with skin laxity, the inferior border of the mandible becomes indistinct, often blending straight into the contour of the neck or nearly so. This shape needs to be projected blending superiorly and anteriorly into surrounding tissues but leaving a sharply defined edge inferiorly. Crosshatching with vertical threads of filler along the ramus and horizontal threads along the body with a 2-cm area of overlap at the angle is a good start to building the desired shape. Depressions along the body posterior to the jowl are occasionally seen and respond to linear threading or occasionally several small superficial–deep pillars or blebs of filler. Jawline correction, properly balanced with cheek contour, can enhance substantially the beauty of the youthful face and contribute significantly to rejuvenation of the aging face.

TEMPLES

The temples deepen with aging, presumably from a reduction in volume of the temporal fat pad and eventually the temporalis muscle itself. The overlying skin is often quite thin and underlying vasculature may be readily visible. This leads to great potential for visible lumps and irregularities, as well as emphasizing the need to avoid overcorrection, which creates an unnatural bulging in this area. The dilution of either HA or CaHa fillers to create a thinner material that readily spreads across the tissue plane makes it easier to obtain an even result. There is guidance about preferred dilutions for this off-label technique. Generally, the dilution adds one-half as much saline or local anesthesia to up to 2 times as much. This author most commonly uses a 1:1 dilution, allowing treatment of both temples with a single syringe of material or sometimes less if the depression is modest. The injection is done as a bolus in 1 or 2 areas followed by massage to smoothly distribute the material. The skin is tented up before insertion of the needle to facilitate placement into the subcutaneous space or deep to the superficial temporal fascia as desired. Accessory longitudinal threading can be performed along the medial portions of the temple to augment any depressions extending into the supraorbital area.

LOWER EYELIDS

Aging in the lower eyelid produces a constellation of changes, each of which is best addressed by a different treatment modality. Although deepening of the tear trough and the development of a visible demarcation at the lid–cheek junction can be addressed surgically, HA filler injection provides a rapid, reliable, and relatively durable solution (**Fig. 6**). Owing to thin skin in this area, selection of filler should tend toward HA fillers that are smooth, soft, fully hydrated, and spread through tissues easily (lower viscosity and cohesivity) to avoid visible lumps and unintentional overcorrection. Put another way, in the lids, the best filler is what you see is what you get—or softer and smoother if possible.

Tear trough correction is the most reliable, quickest, and simplest area to treat in the lower lid. Before deciding that the tear trough is an aesthetically objectionable aging change, the patient must be questioned and photographs of the youthful patient reviewed. If the tear trough has deepened, effacing this will create a more rested look. Linear threading or placement of a bleb of material supraperiosteal, followed by mechanical distribution by rolling that material superiorly with a cotton applicator, is this author's preferred technique. If threading, care must be taken to avoid the angular artery at the apex of the trough near the medial canthus. If placing a bleb, there is concern that vascular cannulation would be more likely to result in embolization. Also, a large quantity of HA filler in this thin-skinned area is more likely to

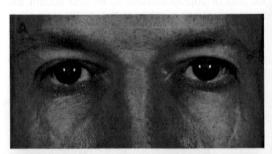
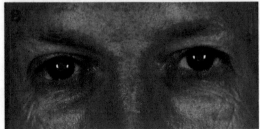

Fig. 6. (*A*) Before treatment. (*B*) At 2 years after correction of the lid cheek junction with a hyaluronic acid filler.

produce a Tyndall effect. Care must also be taken to place the material in the visible depression and not somewhat inferior to it, manifesting a bulge in the upper malar area 1 or 2 weeks later.

The lid–cheek junction can also be corrected but fraught with more risk of ecchymosis. The mid portion usually has several superficial blood vessels. Sometimes, these vessels can be seen at the surface, although they usually coincide with a noticeably depressed portion of the junction that requires correction. Suborbicularis threading of tiny amounts of filler is this author's preferred technique, but often ecchymosis results requiring suspension of the treatment for several minutes to apply gentle but unremitting pressure. Despite this precaution, ecchymosis is likely in this situation. Fortunately, pronounced ecchymosis lasting 1 or 2 weeks is uncommon if the injection technique is gentle and slow. The same is true of the lateral canthal area and the lateral third of the lid cheek junction. Often, the stepoff in this area is rather pronounced, and is occasionally made worse by overly exuberant augmentation of the upper malar area. This needs to be blended, but branches of the zygomaticofacial vessels are easily encountered and rarely visible through the skin surface. This author performs tear trough correction warning of possible ecchymosis, but without undue concern. In the remainder of the lower lid, the author cautions patients to expect at least some ecchymosis. Creasing in the preseptal lid or at the junction of the preseptal and pretarsal portions is common. This can be moderately corrected using suborbicularis fill with tiny threads of injected HA filler or a combination of suborbicularis and subcutaneous fill. Injected volumes are barely discernible, but after settling and blending of the injected filler, significant correction of creasing and crepiness can be obtained. Adding vertical threads for crosshatching can amplify the correction in the lid proper and at the lid–cheek junction.

UPPER EYELIDS/BROWS

The periocular area is anatomically dense. Injection of the upper or lower lid requires a good knowledge of this anatomy and substantial familiarity with the handling properties of the fillers used and a good amount of technical facility. These are not beginner injections or the most commonly performed ones. Despite these challenges, the impact on facial appearance is usually substantial, because this is the part of the face that receives eye contact most of the time during social interactions. These considerations suggest that a provider who is a regular injector should take the trouble to gain proficiency in this area.

Upper lid treatments are infrequent compared with lower lid treatments, but are in some ways less challenging and less risky even if less commonly indicated. The 2 typical treatments are designed to boost the lateral brow and fill upper lid hollowing, whether the result of excessive surgical resection in blepharoplasty, proptosis, or bony architecture of the orbit.

Lateral brow ptosis, if substantial, is best treated with some form of brow lifting. However, like minimal early laxity in the face, early brow ptosis can be minimized by placing small amounts of filler between the soft tissue of the brow and the bony orbital rim. The injection technique involves placing the needle in just lateral to the brow and directing it along the transition zone between the 2 structures mentioned. Short threads or small blebs are placed retrograde as the needle is withdrawn. Less commonly, 1 or 2 small blebs can be placed deep to superficial as a pillar. A denser HA filler or CaHa can be used here. This treatment is best done with moderate expectations and restraint. Small changes are easy to obtain, but the effect is not magnified linearly with more filler.

Upper lid hollowing or skeletonization with a visible orbital rim and hollowing or depression inferior to this but above the pretarsal lid can be camouflaged with hyaluronate filler using a transverse threading technique. Material must be carefully placed because it is difficult to manipulate the material after injection using manual massage, rolling, or other techniques.

NECK, CHEST, AND HANDS

The neck, chest, and hands are areas where thin, sun-damaged skin show fine wrinkling and crepiness. Active dermal response fillers that stimulate substantial amounts of collagen production can be injected in highly diluted form to produce some thickening of the skin over time, blunting the visibility of crepey changes.[6] This is ideally done with CaHa or poly-L-lactic acid. Typical dilutions with CaHa are to a final volume 1.5 to 3 times the starting volume in the syringe.

In the hand, small contour depressions can be corrected with any of the available fillers, including HA, again in diluted form. In the hands, these include features such as the volume loss in between metacarpals, and increased visibility of the veins and tendons. Treatment is performed by placing small blebs of material deep to the skin while taking care not to enter the tendon sheaths or any of the dorsal veins. Injection must be made in multiple places to ensure that the filler ends up in all areas of the hand. Connective tissue septae exist that inhibit spread of the material across the entire dorsum. Vigorous massage for several minutes is then required to distribute the material as evenly as possible.

FOREHEAD/GLABELLA

The glabella forms rhytids that are predominately dynamic in nature and amenable to correction with botulinum toxin injection. However, a component of dermal change or contour depression develops as aging progresses. Small amounts of intradermal HA can provide a more complete correction in these circumstances. Intradermal injection minimizes the risk of possible intravascular injection that would be present if subdermal injection is performed. This author does not believe that use of blunt cannulas eliminates the risk of intravascular injection. Given the proximity in this area to supraorbital and supratrochlear vessels a dermal plane with constant motion, threading and no bleb placement is safer.

Forehead contour, particularly in the supraorbital and lower forehead area, can be modulated using injectable filler. Small depressions above the orbital rim can be filled with a threading technique. Tranverse forehead lines are not readily corrected using currently available injectable fillers. Superficial injection with low viscosity and cohesivity fillers can be cautiously performed but care must be taken to avoid beading and visible overcorrection. For this reason, injection for this indication is not performed commonly.

ACNE SCARS AND TRAUMATIC CONTOUR DEPRESSIONS

Acnes scars and other depressed, tethered scars are treated with intradermal injection with or without subcision. Subcision involves sweeping the bevel of a needle beneath the scar to release the dermis from underlying tissues. This technique can be augmented by additional subdermal fill to prevent the skin from healing back down in a tethered position. Although HA fillers have been used, recent approval of poly methylmethacrylate beads suspended in collagen for treatment of acne scars holds promise for long-lasting correction.[7]

SUMMARY

Judiciously applied, injectable fillers provide an effective solution for a wide range of aesthetic issues. Approved materials after more biocompatible and durable than ever before and future additions are likely to provide even more utility. Outcomes will continue to depend heavily on artistic analysis, anatomic knowledge, and precise injection technique.

REFERENCES

1. Available at: http://www.surgery.org/sites/default/files/2014-Stats.pdf.
2. Wang F, Garza LA, Kang S, et al. In vivo stimulation of de novo collagen production caused by cross-linked hyaluronic acid dermal filler injections in photodamaged human skin. Arch Dermatol 2007;143:155–63.
3. Bass LS, Smith S, Busso M, et al. Calcium hydrolapatite (Radiesse) for treatment of nasolabial folds: Long-term safety and efficacy results. Aesthetic Surgery Journal 2010;30(2):235–8.
4. Sundaram H, Cassuto D. Biophysical characteristics of hyaluronic acid soft-tissue fillers and their relevance to aesthetic applications. Plast Reconstr Surg 2013;132(4 Suppl 2):5S–21S.
5. Rohrich RJ, Pessa JE. The fat compartments of the face: anatomy and clinical implications for cosmetic surgery. Plast Reconstr Surg 2007;119(7):2219–27.
6. Van Loghem J, Yutskovskaya YA, Werschler WP. Calcium hydroxylapatite: over a decade of clinical experience. J Clin Aesthetic Derm 2015;8(1):38–49.
7. Karnik J, Baumann L, Bruce S, et al. A double-blind, randomized, multicenter, controlled trial of suspended polymethylmethacrylate microspheres for the correction of atrophic facial acne scars. J Am Acad Dermatol 2014;71:77–83.

Current Concepts in Filler Injection

Amir Moradi, MD[a],*, Jeffrey Watson, MD[b]

KEYWORDS

- Temple augmentation • Temple rejuvenation • Temple filler • Midface augmentation
- Jawline enhancement and augmentation • Restylane • Radiesse • Juvederm voluma XC

KEY POINTS

- Volumization of the temples is a safe and effective use of dermal fillers to decrease hollowness. This article describes injection technique and outcomes.
- Volumization and enhancement of the midface can restore a youthful look and achieve symmetry. This article addresses placement of the device and injection technique.
- Jawline augmentation can be effective with the correct placement and product or combination of products.

TEMPORAL AUGMENTATION AND REJUVENATION

Treatment Goals and Planned Outcomes

In rejuvenation of the temples, the goal is to obtain a youthful and aesthetic result that is appropriate for each individual, in a safe and effective manner. For example, the temples of an individual with bony structures of the face and thin skin should have more of a concavity than an individual with a rounder face and thicker skin. The challenges that face the injector in this area include vascular structures, muscles of mastication, and emissary and diploic veins of the skull. The skin in this area could be thin in individuals needing treatment; thus, the product used could become visible if not placed appropriately.

Preoperative Planning and Preparation

Selection of an appropriate candidate is based on the trained eye of the injecting physician. Many patients may not be aware of the presence of hollowness in this area and it has to be brought up to them by the treating physician by the use of a mirror or photographs.[1] At times, the treatment of this aesthetic unit is essential for a more balanced and youthful result. Photographs are essential using a superior oblique view (**Fig. 1**). The patient needs to be prepped with an antiseptic solution. This preparation has become more important with observed infection that can occur in the face at times, often months later.[2] One may consider decreasing the viscosity of the filler by using lidocaine. If there are any concerns about causing irregularities in thin-skinned individuals, this dilution is optimal. During the injection, one must plan on transitioning into the surrounding structures. For example, the temporal region transitions into the forehead at the temporal line and, if there is loss of volume medial to this, an optimal aesthetic outcome may necessitate gradual injection medially beyond the temporal line for a smooth transition.

Dr A. Moradi is a board-certified facial plastic surgeon in private practice at Moradi MD in Vista (San Diego County), California. Dr A. Moradi is a paid speaker, investigator, consultant, and advisory board member for Allegan (Dublin, Ireland), Galderma Laboratories (Ft Worth, Texas), and Merz North America (Raleigh, North Carolina). Dr J. Watson reports no disclosures.
[a] Private Practice, 2023 West Vista Way, Suite F, Vista, CA 92083, USA; [b] University of California San Diego Medical Center, 9500 Gilman Drive, Mail Code 0012, San Diego, CA 92093, USA
* Corresponding author.
E-mail address: moradimd@gmail.com

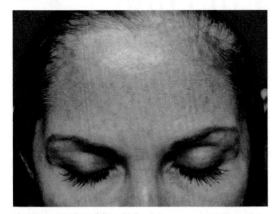

Fig. 1. Superior oblique view.

Patient Positioning

The temporal area is fairly fixed and does not change or move significantly with head position; thus, proper position depends on comfort and ease of injection. This is in contrast with the mid-face and jawline, because these units shift depending on head position from vertical to supine.

Procedural Approach

There are several described techniques for injection in this region.[3] The authors prefer subcutaneous injections owing to safety and ease of augmentation. Patients can be graded using the temporal hollowness grading system (**Table 1**). After delineation of the area to be treated, anesthetic cream is applied and the skin is prepped with an antiseptic solution. The injections are placed in the immediate subcutaneous tissue, between the skin and superficial temporal fascia (**Fig. 2**). The volume per injection is kept at small aliquots of 0.1 mL or less per injection (**Fig. 3**). The skin is massaged after each injection.

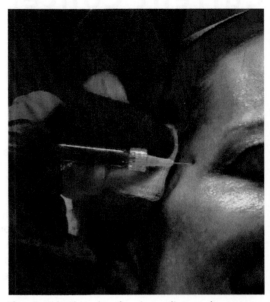

Fig. 2. Injection in the immediate subcutaneous tissue.

Potential Complications and Their Management

Although the first author has never had any significant complications administering this procedure, there are reports of complications, mostly owing to vascular occlusions as a result of injections in this area.[4] Based on a study at one of the first authors practice, the complications or adverse events were defined as any unfavorable or unintended sign, symptom, reaction, or disease associated in time with the use of an investigational

Table 1
Hollowness severity rating scale

Score	Description
4	Severe: very hollow temples. Significant improvement is expected from injectable implant.
3	Moderate: moderately hollow temples. Excellent correction is expected from injectable implant.
2	Mild: shallow hollow temples; minor facial feature. Implant is expected to produce a slight improvement in appearance.
1	Absent: no hollowness.

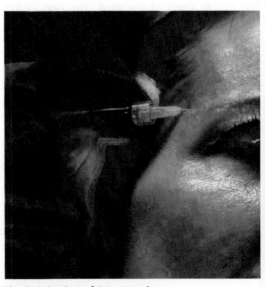

Fig. 3. Injection of 0.1 mL or less.

drug or device. Safety was assessed by evaluating all local and systemic adverse events at all visits as well as in the patient diaries. All adverse events documented by the evaluator and through patient diaries were mild or moderate and resolved by the 2-week follow-up (**Table 2**). One patient noted "hyperpigmentation" in her diary; however, within 2 weeks the mark was completely invisible, and upon questioning the patient, the investigator determined that the adverse event was ecchymosis.

There were 2 instances where a community practitioner contacted one of the authors regarding vascular necrosis in the temporal area. In both cases, the filler was reportedly injected into deep tissues. In both cases, the cardinal signs included transient blanching of the lateral forehead progressing to a reticular pattern, significant pain that was delayed in onset and intensified after several hours of injection, and the appearance of vesicles that were interpreted as an herpetic outbreak. These patients went on to develop necrosis of the superficial dermis with scarring. Both practitioners reported massaging the area once they saw the blanching until the skin turned pink. In the first author's opinion, once a large bolus of the product is infused intraarterially and massaged, it is forced to move distally into the end arterioles. Depending on the particle size, lodging at the corresponding vessel diameter[5] could explain the immediate transient revascularization, followed by the reticular pattern of blanched and purplish skin.

Postprocedural Care

Immediately after the procedure, the patient was asked to apply light pressure for about 5 minutes and then followed with application of ice packs.

Table 2
Adverse events

Adverse Event	n (%)
Bruising	14 (70)
Redness	13 (65)
Tenderness	20 (100)
Pain	16 (80)
Swelling	20 (100)
Hyperpigmentation	1 (5)
Skin irregularities	11 (55)
Headache	15 (75)
Chewing	2 (10)
Jaw ache	1 (5)

All subjects are counseled regarding temporary bumps, bruising, swelling, headaches, and tenderness on mastication.

Rehabilitation and Recovery

All patients are advised to return to their normal daily activities as soon as the injection session is completed. However, patients should be advised to refrain from strenuous exercises for 24 hours to avoid potential swelling and bruising.

Outcomes

In a clinical study,[3] all patients were satisfied with the aesthetic outcome of the procedure. In the first author's treatment of more than 1000 patients with this technique, the rate of dissatisfaction is extremely low (**Figs. 4** and **5**).

MIDFACE AND MALAR AUGMENTATION

Many surgical approaches have been described in the rejuvenation of the midface.[6–8] As the use of facial fillers has progressed, more physicians use fillers to rejuvenate the midface by volumization and restructuring of this facial aesthetic area. It is the authors' belief that the midface is one of the focal points when using facial fillers in aesthetic rejuvenation. In contrast with the temples, where the limits of augmentation are fairly clear owing to its structural boundaries, the midface does not have those clear boundaries. At the Food and Drug Administration's (FDA) request, the facial subregions that could be used to capture treatment, safety, and effectiveness data were defined. Three midface subregions were defined—the zygomaticomalar region, the anteromedial cheek, and the submalar region. Because all outcomes were similar across facial subregions, this paper focuses on results for overall midface volume deficit.[9] Depending on the placement of the filler,

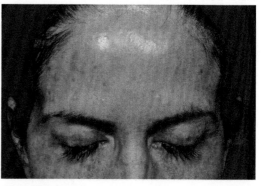

Fig. 4. Baseline.

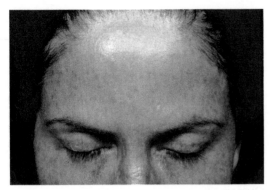

Fig. 5. At 12 months after injection to the temporal region.

the midface prominence and focal point can change as follows:

1. Lateral zygoma (lateral to a line drawn from lateral cantus to oral commissure), increase width of the midface and shift the focal point laterally
2. Midcheek (medial to a line from lateral cantus to oral commissure, above Hinderer's line[10]; anterior projection of the midface, may shift the focal point medially)
3. Submalar (lateral to and a line from lateral cantus to oral commissure and below the Hinderer's line), shift the focal point.

Treatment Goals and Planned Outcomes

The goal in midface augmentation may range from simply restoring the loss of volume to dramatically changing the shape of the midface through placement of the fillers in noninherent locations. Ample time has to be spent interviewing the patient and evaluating his or her facial structures. In the authors' experience, most faces are asymmetrical and usually 1 side of the face appears more youthful than the other. Any such findings must be communicated to the patient. Furthermore, the authors believe that the first step in facial filler augmentation is to use the more youthful side as the template while injecting the contralateral side for symmetry. Once close symmetry is reached, then further injections can be made on both sides to further enhance bilateral facial structures.

Preoperative Planning and Preparation

Once the patient and the physician have decided mutually on a desired outcome, facial photographs must be taken at least in 3 views. These views should include the frontal and bilateral oblique. The authors have often evaluated printed photographs to look for details such as variations in

the height and width of the zygoma and subtle asymmetries in the malar prominence. Differences in the transition from the midface to the surrounding aesthetic units can also be observed photographically. Furthermore, these photographs can help to communicate to the patient subtle findings that may have been missed when viewed in the mirror (**Fig. 6**).

Patient Positioning

The soft tissue structures of the midface are relatively mobile; therefore, the patient's head must be placed in an upright position during evaluation and treatment. Furthermore, this facial structure is 3-dimensional and geometrically complex. Subtle changes can make large visual differences. The physician must be able to move around the treatment chair freely and evaluate the outcome progressively from different viewpoints for a better 3-dimensional outcome.

Procedural Approach

In most cases, injections are started laterally over the periosteum of the zygoma. The authors believe that the zygoma provides a firm and reliable base to lift the midface in a supralateral direction. The injector needs to be cognizant of the entire face and create a natural transition to other surrounding facial aesthetic units in a 3-dimensional fashion.

Potential Complications and Their Management

Most adverse events include swelling and bruising, which usually resolves within 7 to 10 days. The risks and complications associated may include asymmetry and irregularities, infection, skin necrosis, and blindness.

Postprocedural Care

The area treated is massaged thoroughly and the patient is asked to place a cold compress over

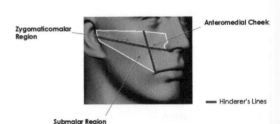

Fig. 6. Three subregions defined in the study. (*From* Jones D, Murphy DK. Volumizing hyaluronic acid filler for midface volume deficit: 2-year results from a pivotal single-blind randomized controlled study. Dermatol Surg 2013;39:1603; with permission.)

the treated area. Furthermore, the patient is asked to call immediately if she or he experiences any unusual pain or changes in the skin color other than the expected tenderness, swelling, and bruising.

Rehabilitation and Recovery

The patient can return to their usual activity by the next day.

Outcomes

The ideal outcome is restoration of a more youthful and attractive midface in harmony with the rest of the facial features.

JAWLINE AUGMENTATION
Treatment Goals and Planned Outcomes

As with any facial region, the proper evaluation and treatment plan is paramount to the creation of a natural, youthful, and more attractive appearance. This region of the face is more difficult to evaluate and treat based on the number of structural variables involved, such as

1. Position and prominence of the mandibular angle
2. Length of the mandible
3. Thickness of the skin and subcutaneous tissue
4. Height, projection, and width of the chin
5. Cervicomental angle.

Preoperative Planning and Preparation

A comprehensive evaluation may include assessment of the thickness of skin and subcutaneous tissues, inherent asymmetries of the face, bony structures, and history of facial procedures and surgeries, among other factors. The injector needs to be well aware of the anatomic structures that are in vicinity of injection sites, such as the parotic gland, masseter muscle, blood vessels, and nerves.

Patient Positioning

The soft tissue surrounding this facial aesthetic unit is relatively mobile and may shift depending on the position of the head and neck. During evaluation and treatment, the patient needs to be at an upright sitting position. The injector needs to be able to move around the treatment chair to view the face from different angles and also be able to visualize the inferior border of the mandible.

Procedural Approach

The authors propose a general guide in contouring the jaw line as described in the pictures. A youthful jawline usually consists of a smooth transition from the mentum transecting an imaginary line parallel to the angle of the auricle adjacent to the tragus. For patients who have a poorly defined bony outline, this topographic guide could be used in creating an aesthetically pleasing jawline.

The objective of this procedure includes achievement of the most optimal aesthetic outcome using the safest and most effective procedure and product. The first author's current product of choice is based on what is needed to accomplish the best aesthetic outcome for a specific individual. Judging from the last decade, future fillers may be even more specific to the intended structural tissues. At the time of the publication of this article, the products of choice include a highly elastic hyaluronic acid such as Juvéderm Voluma XC (Allergan), Perlane (Galderma), and solid particles of calcium hydroxylapatite (Radiesse, Merz). A hybrid mixture of the Radiesse with a hyaluronic acid in varying concentrations depending on the desired aesthetic outcome can also be used. This preference is based on the physical characteristics of these products that provide a firm and sculpted augmentation of this bony structure. Although in most cases either of these products can be used to rejuvenate the jawline, there are cases in which either Juvéderm Voluma XC, Perlane, or Radiesse provides the ideal aesthetic outcome.

Thin skin over well-defined and prominent mandible; need for soft tissue augmentation	Soft tissue augmentation: Compressible filler: as Juvéderm Voluma XC, Perlane
Thick skin and tissue, poorly defined mandibular structure, need for defining the bony structure to support the overlying tissues	Rigid structural augmentation: Incompressible filler: Radiesse
Thick skin and tissue; well-defined mandibular structure	Lifting augmentation: Either product or combination of both

Potential Complications and Their Management

For safety reasons and better aesthetic outcome, small volumes of 0.1 mL or less must be administered per injection point and massaged. With the release of the new formulation of Radiesse with lidocaine, a 27-gauge needle may be used to inject the product. In the past the author has used

0.26 mL of 1% or 2% lidocaine (plain) mixed with 1.5 mL of calcium hydroxylapatite, using a 29-gauge needle to decrease the flow rate and better control the volume injected.

Postprocedural Care

Patients are counseled regarding the swelling, bruising, and pain with mastication. All patients are discharged with a cold compress. They are asked to massage the area twice a day for about 2 to 3 minutes for 3 days.

SUMMARY

Since the introduction of FDA-approved synthetic fillers, the use of these products in facial volumization and restructuring has increased significantly. The demand for nonoperative procedures continues to grow and new devices are constantly evolving. The options for nonoperative volumization and sculpting continue to evolve as more physicians and patients learn and experience the outcomes that fillers can provide.

REFERENCES

1. Moradi A, Shirazi A, Perez V. A guide to temporal fossa augmentation with small gel particle hyaluronic acid dermal filler. J Drugs Dermatol 2011;10(6):673–6.
2. Lowe NJ, Maxwell CA, Patnaik R. Adverse reactions to dermal fillers: review. Dermatol Surg 2005;31(s4):1626–33.
3. Moradi A, Shirazi A, Moradi J. A 12-month, prospective, evaluator-blinded study of small gel particle hyaluronic acid filler in the correction of temporal fossa volume loss. J Drugs Dermatol 2013;12(4):470–5.
4. Narins RS, Jewell M, Rubin M, et al. Clinical conference: management of rare events following dermal fillers—focal necrosis and angry red bumps. Dermatol Surg 2006;32(3):426–34.
5. Kim DW, Yoon ES, Ji YH, et al. Vascular complications of hyaluronic acid fillers and the role of hyaluronidase in management. J Plast Reconstr Aesthet Surg 2011;64(12):1590.
6. Ramirez OM. Three-dimensional endoscopic midface enhancement: a personal quest for the ideal cheek rejuvenation. Plast Reconstr Surg 2002;109(1):329–40.
7. Hamra ST. The zygorbicular dissection in composite rhytidectomy: an ideal midface plane. Plast Reconstr Surg 1998;102(5):1646–57.
8. Terino EO, Edward M. The magic of mid-face three-dimensional contour alterations combining alloplastic and soft tissue suspension technologies. Clin Plast Surg 2008;35(3):419–50.
9. Jones D, Murphy DK. Volumizing hyaluronic acid filler for midface volume deficit: 2-year results from a pivotal single-blind randomized controlled study. Dermatol Surg 2013;39:1–11.
10. Carruthers J, Rzany B, Sattler G, et al. Anatomic guidelines for augmentation of the cheek and infraorbital hollow. Dermatol Surg 2012;38(7 Pt 2):1223–33.

Index

Moving?

Make sure your subscription moves with you!

To notify us of your new address, find your **Clinics Account Number** (located on your mailing label above your name), and contact customer service at:

Email: journalscustomerservice-usa@elsevier.com

800-654-2452 (subscribers in the U.S. & Canada)
314-447-8871 (subscribers outside of the U.S. & Canada)

Fax number: 314-447-8029

Elsevier Health Sciences Division
Subscription Customer Service
3251 Riverport Lane
Maryland Heights, MO 63043

*To ensure uninterrupted delivery of your subscription, please notify us at least 4 weeks in advance of move.

ELSEVIER

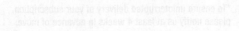

Printed and bound by CPI Group (UK) Ltd, Croydon, CR0 4YY

03/10/2024

01040381-0005